Mental Health Workbook for Men

Mental Health Workbook

FOR MEN

Exercises to Improve Your Emotional, Psychological, and Social Well-Being

DAVID KHALILI, LMFT

ROCKRIDGE
PRESS

First Rockridge Press trade paperback edition 2023

Rockridge Press and the Rockridge Press logo are trademarks or registered trademarks of Callisto Media Inc. and/or its affiliates in the United States and other countries and may not be used without written permission.

For general information on our other products and services, please contact our Customer Care Department within the United States at (866) 744-2665, or outside the United States at (510) 253-0500.

Paperback ISBN: 978-1-63878-256-8 | eBook ISBN: 978-1-63878-402-9

Manufactured in the United States of America

Interior and Cover Designer: Lisa Forde
Art Producer: Stacey Stambaugh
Editor: Mo Mozuch
Production Editor: Rachel Taenzler
Production Manager: Riley Hoffman

Illustrations © Alexey Lesik/Shutterstock (fractal background)

10 9 8 7 6 5 4 3 2 1 0

To my father, nephew, and son. Three important influences on how I see, hold, and challenge masculinity. To Alyson, thank you for your many lessons and modeling of mindfulness.

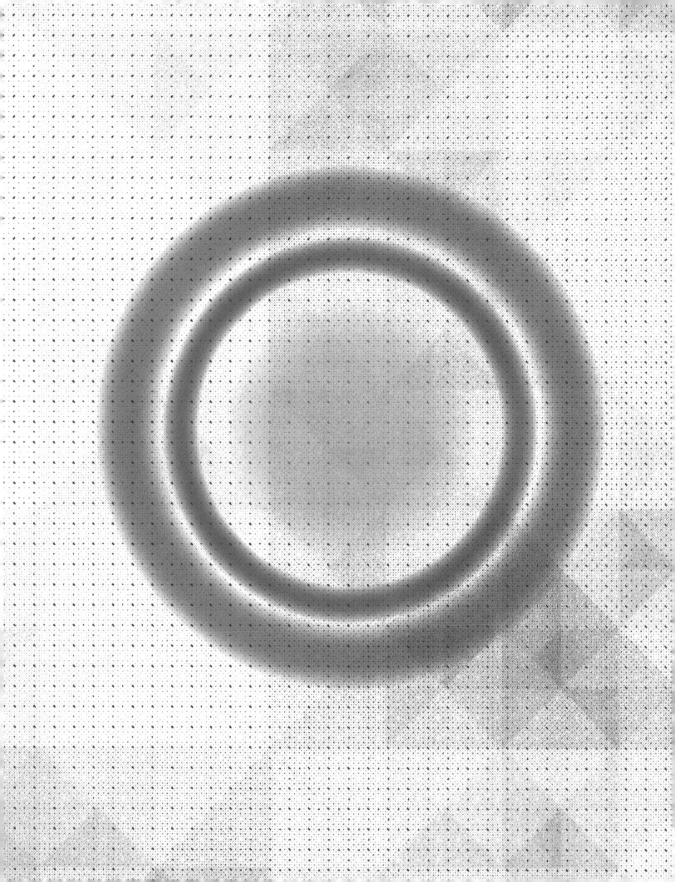

Contents

Introduction

Welcome to the *Mental Health Workbook for Men*. I'm David Khalili, a licensed marriage and family therapist, and board-certified sexologist. As a man and a therapist, I have worked with and examined how masculinity, gendered expectations, and stereotypes impact men's mental health. While growing up as a first-generation American-born boy, I saw and experienced how various cultures expected their boys and men to hide their emotions. I aim to show you that strength means facing your emotions, seeing them through their process, and developing various skills to cope with and celebrate the human experience.

To model honesty and validate others, I admit I'm not as accepting and mindful of my emotions and experiences as I aspire to be. It's not always easy, but I've found it's worthwhile to work on it over time. Remember that mental health, like physical health, will be something to attend to and nurture throughout your life.

Why dedicate an entire workbook to the mental health of men? As you'll see throughout the book, rigid masculine stereotypes have created a narrow range of acceptable emotions for men. For example, you may have heard that men are "only allowed to be horny, happy, or angry." In *The Will to Change*, philosopher bell hooks wrote about how men can access emotions, show love, and receive love through rejecting patriarchal standards. "Learning to wear a mask (that word already embedded in the term 'masculinity') is the first lesson in patriarchal masculinity that a boy learns. He learns that his core feelings cannot be expressed if they do not conform to the acceptable behaviors sexism defines as male." This emotional hold makes it socially risky for men to express themselves or ask for help.

Regardless of your assigned sex at birth, this workbook is designed to help all men, including trans men, navigate mental health and address issues that are particularly pressing for men these days. Elements of this book can be helpful for nonbinary folks who have experienced male socialization and feel like they can benefit from this perspective.

Let's cover the difference between mental health and mental illness to ensure you're clear on what is impacting you and what we are addressing. Just because your mental health isn't well doesn't mean you have a mental illness. Mental health involves balancing emotional, psychological, and social needs and being able to engage in daily activities. On the other hand, mental illness is a cluster of diagnosable symptoms that can include trouble regulating your mood, distorted thinking, issues with your behavior, and significant problems in your relationships.

Throughout the book, you'll have a chance to use a variety of exercises structured from evidence-based modalities like mindfulness-based stress reduction, acceptance and commitment therapy (ACT), and positive psychology. The book is designed to be followed from cover to cover, yet each exercise is accessible independently. What's important is that you take your time, be nice to yourself, and be ready to commit to some action aligned with your values and needs.

How to Use This Workbook

Think of this workbook more as a journey or a process rather than a casual read. You deserve to take the time and energy to learn about yourself and how you operate in the world. The hope for this book is that you get to develop a deeper relationship with yourself by learning how emotions, thoughts, and social factors impact mental health. Furthermore, you'll understand how you interact with these three factors.

This book is not meant to be a replacement for therapy or other forms of healing. This is intended to be a supplement. Over fifty exercises in this book are designed to help you learn about yourself and develop new skills to improve your mental health. Not all of these exercises will be right for you or work in your favor. However, please keep track of the ones that work well for you so you can easily access them when needed. It may also be useful to look at the exercises that felt helpful and see if there's a pattern or reason why they stood out to you.

The goal of this book is not to cure, fix, or give you what you need overnight. Instead, the goal is to help you continually move a few percentage points toward happiness and well-being while accepting and working through tough times. For example, in the book *10% Happier*, Dan Harris shares how mindfulness doesn't cure your problems, but it makes you more reflective in how you respond to your concerns. This framing can be constructive because it takes off the perfectionistic pressure to get everything right and to do things quickly.

You deserve consistent, loving, and caring exploration. Let yourself get into a flow with this work and schedule a regular time one to three times a week to sink into this book. After you finish, you may realize that you still want to use that time for further self-work. If that's the case, continue to protect that time for yourself.

Offering a queer perspective, I share exercises to encourage pushing your understanding of masculinity and rigid gender norms. For those who have transitioned, you have undoubtedly considered your gender and gendered expectations throughout your life. I hope these exercises offer a new space to deepen your self-compassion and understanding.

Develop a good relationship with this book. What does that mean? Don't toss the book on the table and groan when you work on the exercises. Instead, make an active choice to approach this workbook in a way that will most benefit you. You're the main person this will benefit, so you might as well make it worth your time.

The workbook uses frameworks from evidence-based modalities like ACT, mindfulness, and positive psychology. As you'll see in the book, these modalities work wonderfully with the emotional, psychological, and social aspects of mental health. An eclectic approach, which picks and chooses the best techniques from different modalities, treats the whole person.

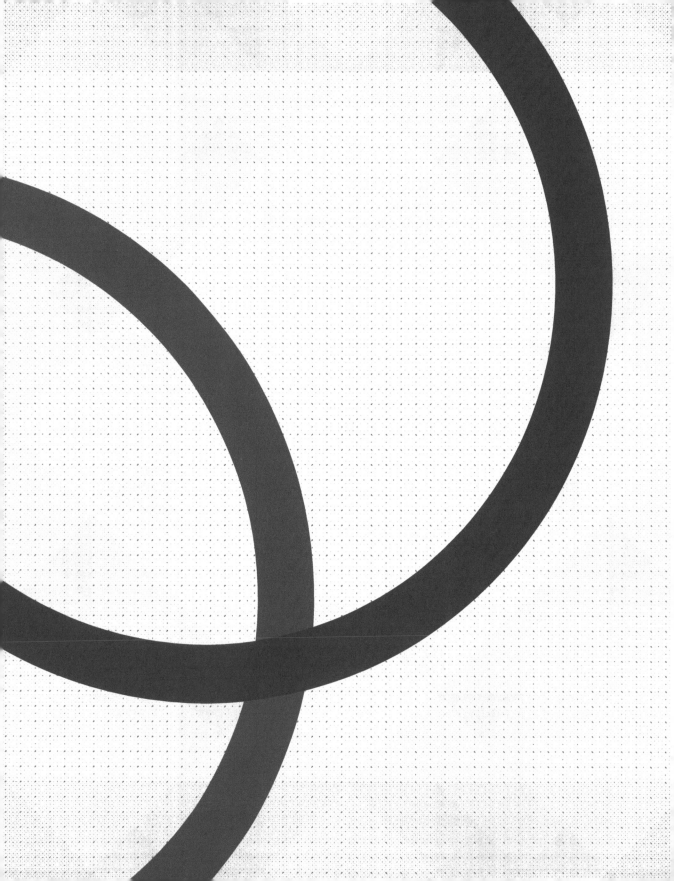

CHAPTER ONE

MENTAL HEALTH AND WELLNESS

> *Understanding, accepting, and improving my*
> *mental health is a strength. Seeking help*
> *and support shows my willingness to be honest*
> *with my values, needs, and integrity.*

What Is Mental Health?

Mental health is a complex collection of emotional, psychological, and social factors. Emotional mental health involves an unattached awareness of your feelings, knowledge of triggers, and acceptance of the breadth and depth of your emotional life. Elements of psychological mental health include knowledge of your trauma and stress responses and how they interact with your body and mind, practicing elements of mindfulness, and making healthy choices. Finally, social factors include the cultivation and maintenance of healthy, supportive, and mutually facilitative (you make time for each other) relationships. Furthermore, your mental health benefits from knowing your attachment styles, holding yourself accountable, and setting and maintaining healthy boundaries.

These factors can impact how we act and react to things like our feelings, life stressors, and interpersonal relationships. By navigating how we interact with, manage, and accept these factors, we can work toward improved mental health.

Working on your mental health also involves allowing yourself to grow. In order to grow, you need to admit to yourself that your past choices may no longer work for you.

Balancing emotional, social, and psychological elements of mental health and holding oneself accountable may not be a barrier for all guys. However, one or a combination of those are common obstacles for men due to stigma and social pressure around mental health and getting support.

Environmental Factors

When working on your mental health, it's essential to acknowledge the influences outside of yourself that affect your well-being. If we don't recognize these factors, we're essentially lying to ourselves by giving an inaccurate picture of what is and isn't our responsibility and within our control. By accurately and explicitly naming the environmental factors in your life that impact your mental health, you can then identify what is within your control to make changes for positive growth. Otherwise, you'll sit there wholly overwhelmed, thinking it should all be within your power to change when you really only have a certain amount of control.

As a man, you may have been raised to believe that you should handle most things on your own, and that seeking help is weak. You probably developed an unconscious habit of not even recognizing when you could use help, let alone asking for it. In *The Will to Change,* bell hooks writes, "To indoctrinate boys into the rules of patriarchy, we force them to feel pain and to deny their feelings." This tension and paradox is a social pressure that harms many lives, not just male-identifying folks.

Work stress often causes many environmental issues in a man's life. Although women make up a large portion of burnout statistics, men are not that far behind. Many men feel overwhelmed and stuck at a job that provides little meaning, but the pressure to not voice frustrations can leave them feeling isolated.

Global political turmoil, rapidly accelerating climate change, and the twenty-four-hour news cycle can also leave you spinning, dysregulated, and with few actionable steps within your control. As we'll see later, there are various ways to manage environmental stressors. But first, let's break down the difference between mental *health* and mental *illness.*

Mental Health vs. Mental Illness

When thinking about mental health, it's important to recognize that it involves multiple aspects of your life, some in and some and out of your control. Mental health includes:

- Understanding yourself and your body

- Feeling the breadth and depth of emotions

- Coping with life stressors

- Holding yourself equally to others, not better or worse

- Social and community support

Mental health does not mean having complete control over your life or your reactions. Mental health is not a static state. It's something you attend to, understand, and cultivate throughout your life. You do "the work" by continually examining yourself, your actions/reactions, and your interactions with others. Using skills like self-awareness and detached witnessing, which we'll go over later, you can label your thoughts and feelings as they happen.

At this point in the book, I remind you that we're talking about a *process* of self-improvement and identifying ideal goals. These are goals to strive *toward* and not something you flip a switch to achieve. If that were possible, you would have done it by now. So, give yourself the grace to be in the process of learning and developing.

When we discuss *mental illness*, we refer to illnesses or disorders related to genetic issues, neurochemical imbalances, personality disorders, and environmental issues like childhood abuse, other forms of trauma, and substance abuse. Depending on which privileges and resiliencies you hold, you may be more or less susceptible due to environmental factors that increase stress and trauma. Certain mental illnesses, such as schizophrenia, are not trauma-related and, unfortunately, are not curable at the time of this writing. Others are the result of chronic childhood trauma like abuse or neglect. There's no way to undo the trauma, but you can work to understand how it's impacted you and create a personalized set of skills to help you through overwhelming moments.

For those with moderate to severe mental illness diagnoses, you may find that this book lacks depth and focus for your distinct symptoms and diagnoses. However, this book will cover the breadth of mental health among men, so if you're looking for a more specific focus, please look at other workbooks or consult a mental health professional.

Common Mental Health Concerns for Men

Men struggle with various mental health concerns, including depression, anxiety, anger, and burnout. Here are some that we'll be covering throughout the book.

Depression and depressive episodes. A recent study found that 30 percent of men have experienced a period of depression in their life, one in four have sought help from a medical professional, and American men are four times as likely to die by suicide than women. Although depression is sometimes related to an imbalance of neurochemicals, it is also acutely associated with a loss or trauma. For marginalized men, it can result from discrimination and harassment.

Anxiety. Anxiety is a normal and healthy reaction to stressful situations. It serves as a warning system for us to be aware of stress or danger. Anxiety becomes an issue when the "warning system" inaccurately defines what is a stressor or a threat. Physical anxiety symptoms include increased heart rate, sweaty palms, digestive issues, irritability, and difficulty sleeping. Psychological symptoms can include racing thoughts, worst-case thinking, all-or-nothing thinking, and an inability to focus.

Anger and irritability. Anger is a complex emotion that is often treated and addressed without subtlety. You'll see in later exercises that you will be instructed to tune in to your anger rather than push it aside to get a nuanced understanding. Unmanaged anger isn't just harmful to relationships and others; it can be harmful to you. Repeated stress and anger increase hormones like cortisol and adrenaline, which negatively impact heart health.

Pressure to perform. The pressure to perform exists in many domains. It shows up in work, school, finances, and sex. The pressure to perform creates a heightened expectation in a particular way that may not be realistic. In these moments, you benefit from getting an accurate understanding of the expectations, your capacity, and how to communicate any needs or boundaries.

Burnout. Burnout can look like apathy, anxiety, tense muscles, quick temper, or brain fog. These are all ways your mind and body tell you that you are tapped out. In 2019, the World Health Organization made burnout an internationally recognized disease and labeled it an "occupational phenomenon." Burnout has also become four times more common since the beginning of the COVID-19 pandemic.

Substance abuse and addiction. Men are more likely than women to suffer from substance misuse and abuse, and there is an even higher likelihood for trans men. However, women are more likely to seek support for their addiction. Men and trans men often avoid medical or therapeutic support due to social pressure to "solve it on their own" or real or feared discrimination.

Loneliness and isolation. Loneliness in men is correlated with cardiovascular disease and stroke and is seen as one of the reasons why some men attempt suicide. Over their life, many men focus more on building financial stability and career success and less on building and maintaining relationships. They go from having "blood brothers" to Hungry-Man dinners. Although career success is needed for financial stability, emotional currency is vital for your overall well-being.

Unresolved trauma. Trauma left untreated can show up as flashbacks, sudden rage, quickly changing emotions, depression, nightmares, and difficulty in work and relationships. You may think of trauma in men as only related to violence or war. However, early childhood abuse or neglect trauma can have profoundly damaging effects on men if left untreated. Frequently denying treatment can be associated with a stereotyped expectation that boys or men need to "man up" or get over something. However, resolving trauma strengthens you because you gain higher self-awareness and develop healthier coping skills.

WHAT STOOD OUT TO YOU?

An essential component of this workbook, and working on yourself, is building the practice of self-awareness. Meditation, journaling, therapy, and painting are examples of techniques of self-awareness. So, let's start here by checking in on the categories we just discussed.

Using the scales below, indicate where you fall in each category. Take the time to consider if you're entirely unaffected, overwhelmed, or somewhere in between with each one.

Not a concern ——> Overwhelming

Category	1	2	3	4	5
1. Depression:	1	2	3	4	5
2. Anxiety:	1	2	3	4	5
3. Anger:	1	2	3	4	5
4. Pressure to perform:	1	2	3	4	5
5. Burnout:	1	2	3	4	5
6. Substance abuse/addiction:	1	2	3	4	5
7. Loneliness and isolation:	1	2	3	4	5
8. Unresolved trauma:	1	2	3	4	5
9. Imposter syndrome:	1	2	3	4	5
10. Lack of boundaries:	1	2	3	4	5
11. Impulsive/high-risk behaviors:	1	2	3	4	5

It can be useful to occasionally revisit this exercise to see if these concerns have changed over time. You may also consider connecting coping strategies learned later in this book with the aforementioned concerns.

> *I'm not the worst. I'm not the best. I don't have to be either. Encountering the breadth and depth of emotions is part of the human experience and not something to avoid.*

WALID'S SAD TRACKER

Walid looked at himself in the mirror one morning and thought, ***Woof, you look sad.*** He realized he'd been feeling sad for a while. Later that day, he mentioned his sadness to a friend, who suggested he track his mood to check for any patterns. Walid felt a surge of readiness and told his friend he'd commit to checking in every day for a year. His friend softly smiled and suggested he try for a week or two to get the rhythm and go from there. This bite-size chunk of time helped Walid get a taste of the habit. Limiting how much time he spent on the routine helped him focus on checking in rather than worrying about keeping the practice up.

Setting a reminder every morning for two weeks, Walid approached this experiment with appropriate expectations about how much it would help him. Tracking his mood wasn't going to make or break his sadness. Instead, this information gathering would help him learn what level of care he may need.

Before Walid finished the two weeks, he could tell how consistently sad he truly felt. He sighed with a mixture of relief and chagrin. Depression was a familiar visitor, and he had hoped it would have stopped showing up by now. He pulled out his phone to call his doctor to discuss treatment options. After the call, he put on his calendar to play basketball with friends three times a week. From his previous self-work, he knew what coping mechanisms worked best when depressed.

Benefits of Good Mental Health

In moments of good mental health, you find ease in balancing the three dimensions of mental health mentioned previously. Emotionally, psychologically, and socially, you are attuned and aligned. In this attunement, you are also able to understand who you are and *how* you are. You can identify your values, needs, boundaries, and ways of relating. "Good mental health" doesn't mean complete control over yourself and your emotions, but it includes an awareness of what you are feeling and thinking. In that awareness, you can create a buffer to consider your thoughts and feelings as information passing within you, but not necessarily facts you need to react to or engage with.

Another perk of emotional wellness is learning to connect physical sensations to emotions. For example, when you can understand that a rushing feeling in your chest and neck is often associated with anger, you can work to ground yourself. Through psychological well-being, you can understand how your thoughts typically work, what patterns they tend to follow, and how your past experiences and traumas inform your thoughts and feelings. You can be curious about your thoughts and not treat them immediately as facts you need to react to. You can understand and accept that it's healthy to feel various emotions. You can challenge yourself and understand different perspectives on one experience. You can know that you don't have to agree with something to accept that it exists or that it is your reality. For example, you can accept that healthy relationships have ups and downs, even though you may not like it when you're experiencing the downs.

Good mental health also includes improved relationships through understanding your own needs, values, and boundaries and directly communicating them when needed. The social benefits of good mental health include having a community that meets your social needs. Having such also helps you take and accept feedback from others without defensiveness or resentment. Based on the description above, what areas of your mental health feel fulfilled, and what areas deserve more attention?

Mental and Physical Health

While growing up, many boys are falsely given two paths to take: physical health or good grades. They can either be a jock or a nerd, a swim captain or theater kid, a basketball star or a debate team standout. This false dichotomy creates an unnecessary divide between physical and mental skills, as if they couldn't possibly coexist. Finding a balance of mental and physical health is significant for each to function well. It isn't easy to have reasonable mental health without physical health.

Physical health doesn't just mean exercise. It also includes avoiding environmental factors such as:

- Smoking cigarettes
- Alcohol misuse and abuse
- Work stress
- Sleep issues
- Pollution
- Childhood trauma
- Climate change
- Lack of consistent safety (relationship, family, community aggression or violence)

These issues impact your mental health for a variety of reasons. Some concerns, like pollution, substance abuse, and cigarettes, have a chemical impact on your body and mind. Others are related to psychological and physiological effects, like heightened cortisol due to repeated exposure to violence in the home or community.

Harmful male stereotypes directly link to men's imbalance of physical and mental health. Men are socialized to hide their pain to honor the patriarchy (hooks, 2011). By hiding their pain, they show that they agree and uphold the expectation for men to suffer silently. They deny themselves the chance to heal and to stop stress and toxins from overwhelming them. Some examples of the effects of harmful male stereotypes are:

- Internalizing the phrase "walk it off"
- High-risk behavior like binge drinking
- Avoiding medical care
- Not talking about emotions
- Awkwardness reaching out to friends

What is within your control to work toward improved mental health?

Modalities for Treatment

Mental health is a vast topic that spans many different areas of our lives. Whether discussing mental health in terms of our overall well-being or looking specifically at treatments for conditions such as anxiety and depression, finding the right approach can be overwhelming. In this section, I will cover three approaches to mental health treatment: mindfulness, acceptance and commitment therapy (ACT), and positive psychology. Then we'll explore each approach and consider why it might be a good fit for you or someone you know.

This workbook uses evidence-based approaches to increase the chances that the exercises will be effective for you. Evidence-based practices are therapeutic interventions tested and proven through scientific and academic studies, often repeated in multiple studies to show how effective they can be. However, it's important to note that many evidence-based practices were based on research done with white, straight, middle-class folks. To address a more inclusive audience, I have worked to adapt these exercises to incorporate queer theory, critical race theory, and feminist approaches. I firmly believe incorporating these theories with evidence-based practices can improve your chances of undoing internalized harmful male stereotypes.

As you learn more and take on practices and exercises based on these modalities, consider how they do or do not align with your values. For example, are there elements from your culture or family that you can incorporate into these evidence-based practices?

Let's take a quick look at which modalities will be used.

Mindfulness

Mindfulness is a process of being able to healthily detach yourself from your emotions and thoughts. You engage in a subject-object relationship with yourself and your thoughts and feelings. Your thoughts and feelings are the objects, and you are the subject. What we know as mindfulness today originates from four different mindfulness practices: Buddhist, Indian, Tibetan, and Burmese. In the 1960s, a researcher and psychologist named Jon Kabat-Zinn created mindfulness-based stress reduction, which is a practice of using mindfulness to focus on your thoughts and feelings, using acceptance and meditation for grounding practices. The purpose of mindfulness is exactly that: to be mindful of the present moment and work on accepting reality for what it is. It sounds way easier than it is, but it's worth the effort. Research on mindfulness shows that it can be helpful for issues such as stress, grief, anxiety, chronic pain, and trauma. You'll see mindfulness used in various exercises and prompts throughout this workbook to help guide you through noticing your thoughts and feelings without reacting to them right away.

Acceptance and Commitment Therapy

You've probably heard of cognitive behavioral therapy (CBT) but may not be familiar with acceptance and commitment therapy. ACT is a relatively new type of cognitive behavioral therapy that is gaining in popularity. ACT focuses on helping people accept their thoughts and feelings rather than pushing them away like other modalities. ACT follows through on action by encouraging you to commit to living a meaningful life according to your values. Unlike CBT, which focuses on changing problematic thoughts and behaviors, ACT helps people accept themselves as they are. This acceptance can be helpful for those who find themselves stuck in negative thought patterns or have difficulty regulating their emotions. By accepting that "negative" experiences and emotions are part of the human condition, you learn to work with them. ACT can be a valuable tool for anyone who wants to live a more fulfilling life.

ACT follows six fundamental tenets:

- Defusion
- Acceptance
- Contact with the present moment
- The Observing Self
- Values
- Committed action

To learn more about these tenets and to take a deeper dive into ACT, I recommend checking out the *Acceptance and Commitment Therapy Journal* by Dr. Josie Valderrama.

Positive Psychology

There are a lot of misconceptions about positive psychology and the nature of the treatment style. Positive psychology is not simply "looking at the brighter side"—it focuses on a person's strengths or positive characteristics and builds up from there, rather than fixating on a "weakness" or "flaw" to fix and push away.

Psychologist Martin Seligman founded the theory and practice of positive psychology. Seligman gained fame in 1967 after publishing his work on learned helplessness. Learned helplessness is when people or animals feel helpless to avoid negative situations after repeated experiences of their autonomy being ignored or overruled. An example would be a student doing poorly in his science classes and therefore believing he's "just not good at science."

This workbook will incorporate positive psychology to identify your strengths and build from there. Think of your existing strengths as the foundation for the new skills you will gain from your work in this process. Furthermore, using the concept of learned helplessness, you will be given a chance to challenge any self-narratives that have held you back, such as, "I suck at math," or, "No one cares about me."

HECTOR'S ANXIOUS ATTACHMENT

Hector was upset that his boyfriend was leaving on another work trip. During the days leading up to the trip, he made judgmental remarks about his boyfriend's job and choices. He realized that this was a pattern every time his boyfriend left for a trip.

With some embarrassment, Hector approached his boyfriend to apologize for losing his cool before every work trip. His boyfriend was visibly annoyed and said he was "used to it, and now I just tune out your tantrums." Hector felt a twinge of pain in his stomach. It was part shame and part anxiety. He realized this pattern must be more of an issue than he was aware of.

He went to a longtime friend for support. Hector's friend related that he too had an anxious attachment style that made separation from his partner difficult. Through therapy, his friend could connect this experience to his childhood, when his alcoholic mother was inconsistently emotionally present. Hearing this experience set off a big alarm for Hector. He remembered his father's issue with alcohol and how it impacted the whole family. Hector took to journaling to flesh out his thoughts and recognized that his father's alcoholism made him emotionally unavailable, making Hector anxious and upset. Now, when Hector anticipates long periods of unavailability, he goes back to his child self and tries to protest before his partner is unavailable. This is true even though his partner doesn't have an issue with drinking like his father did. Later that week in therapy, Hector shared his thoughts and told his therapist that he wanted to focus on his attachment style in his sessions.

Measuring and Tracking Progress

When it comes to our physical health and fitness, many of us like to measure and track our progress. This helps us see how we're doing and whether we're making improvements over time. It can be a great way to stay motivated and on track with our goals. But what about when it comes to your mental health? Do you ever take the time to measure and track your progress in that area? If not, now is the time to start, because tracking your mental health can be just as important as monitoring your physical health. It can even help you prevent or manage mental health issues down the road.

You'll have opportunities to track and check your progress and process throughout the book. But first, let's talk about how to approach tracking progress.

When looking at your progress, take some time to reflect on the big picture. Focusing too closely on day-to-day changes can disappoint you with the seemingly slow and mundane pacing. However, you can witness progress over time with patience and a shift in your perspective.

It's easy to look back at your past and feel embarrassed at your former self. Be gracious to yourself when you remember acts, thoughts, or choices you made in the past. Acknowledge why you made those choices and how they were likely adaptive to your environment. At this point, it's essential to acknowledge your commitment to making the necessary changes for your betterment.

Consider reminders on your calendar, asking a friend or coworker to be an accountability buddy, or using an app like stickK to help you stay consistent in your progress. If you are choosing someone in your life as an accountability buddy, consider someone who shares this type of self-work as an interest. Through consistent and compassionate accountability checks, you'll be able to develop a sustainable and healthy relationship with understanding and improving yourself.

> *Perfectionism won't protect me against uncomfortable thoughts about myself. I can accept that I am not perfect. My imperfections are part of what makes me who I am.*

LET'S SET GOALS

Based on what you've read in this chapter, and your results from the exercise on page 6, take some time to think about appropriate goals for yourself while using this workbook.

What are some mental health concerns that you'd like to begin or continue addressing in this workbook? You can use the common issues section (page 4) as a reference.

Mental Health Concern 1: _____

Mental Health Concern 2: _____

Mental Health Concern 3: _____

What goals might you have associated with the concerns you listed?

Goal 1: _____

Goal 2: _____

Goal 3: _____

Take a moment and think through your goals. Write out what it would look like to complete these goals. An example would be if you wanted to feel less anxious at night, then the observable part of that goal could be *Get seven to eight hours of sleep two or more days a week.* Using the space provided, write out measurable and observable goals related to your concerns.

Metrics for Goal 1:

_____

_____

_____

Metrics for Goal 2:

_____

_____

_____

Metrics for Goal 3:

_____

_____

_____

How will you hold yourself accountable to these goals (e.g., phone app, friend, calendar reminders, etc.)?

_____

_____

_____

_____

_____

_____

_____

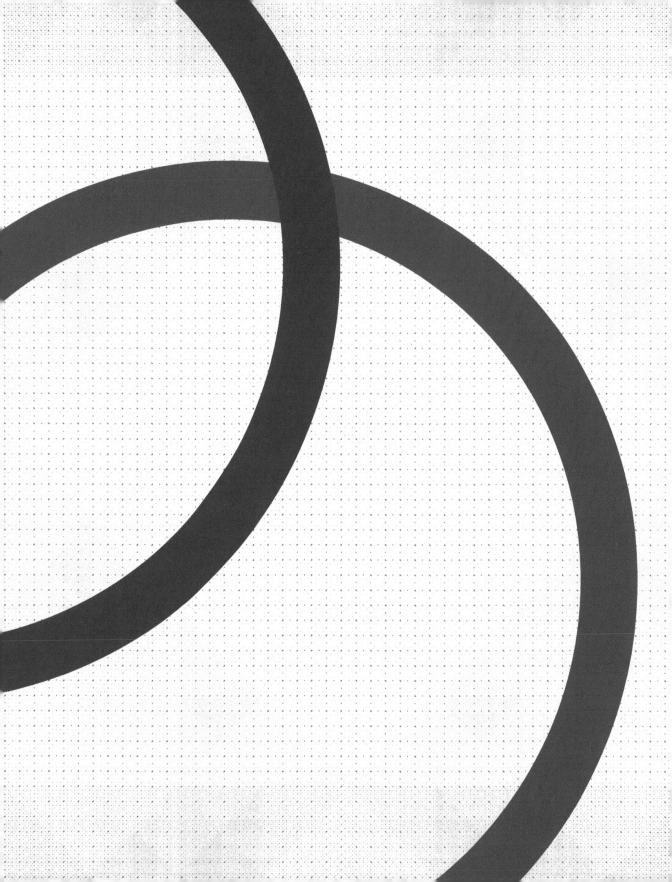

CHAPTER TWO

EMOTIONS AND MENTAL HEALTH

> *It takes strength to step outside my comfort zone.*
> *Vulnerability and connection with*
> *myself and others are worth the discomfort.*

How You Feel

Marco was a standard twenty-six-year-old professional who worked sixty hours a week and drank all weekend. He felt fine throughout his week, but people often asked him if he was okay. He could never figure out what others saw in him that made them worry. His drinking habit started with telling himself "I just **want** to relax," which later led to "I **need** to blow off steam." However, over time, he began to admit that he would either end up sobbing or enraged when drunk. He couldn't predict which end of the emotional spectrum he'd land on when drinking.

The unpredictability of his emotions made him realize he needed to see a therapist specializing in substance abuse. Marco wanted to understand his relationship with alcohol. In his therapeutic work, he realized how much distance he tried to get from his emotions. He was avoiding something by working endless hours throughout the week and dissociating through booze on the weekends.

Marco discovered that he learned through childhood that boys and men shouldn't express their emotions, especially fear. However, Marco has a lot of anxiety. Combining his anxious state with condemning talking about feelings, he was left with a perpetual motion machine of fear and solitude. The excessive work was a strategy to keep his anxiety at bay while also falling in line with capitalist and toxic masculine expectations to show his worth through productivity and financial gain.

Drinking on the weekends was socially acceptable, especially for "hard workers" because they "deserved it."

Through practice sitting with strong emotions for consecutively longer periods, Marco learned and developed more comfort in pushing through gender norms and opening up emotionally to those he trusted.

Does any of Marco's story sound familiar?

In this chapter, we'll cover how emotions work, define various feelings, and explore your relationship with them in more depth.

The Science of Your Emotions

Most of us know the basic emotions. Happiness, sadness, love, and hate are all familiar concepts. But what exactly is happening in our brains when we experience these emotions? And why do we feel them in the first place?

Emotions orchestrate how we feel and experience our environment and are influenced by our physiology and the external world. Our limbic system is the emotional part of the brain. This system interacts with and controls our first wave of emotional responses. We can effectively navigate our lives and relationships with our wide array of emotional responses.

We use our emotions to appraise our environments and release feel-good hormones like dopamine in "good" situations and cortisol or adrenaline in "bad" situations. As you've likely picked up so far, a critical part of your mental health journey is to educate yourself and understand how your emotions work while not judging yourself. Knowing what releases these neurochemicals in your life can help your mental health.

For those with a neurochemical imbalance, traumatic brain injury, or a history of trauma, their limbic system can have difficulty staying regulated. However, through therapy, medication, and other forms of treatment, they can work to adjust their brain chemistry to help find a balance that works for them.

We often think our emotions only operate from our brains. However, there is growing evidence that our gut and gut health are just as important for our emotional health. Ninety-five percent of our serotonin is manufactured in our gut, with other research showing vast improvements in emotional health through anti-inflammatory diets. Does this mean you'll cure your depression through kale? Nope. But it gives credence to treating emotional and mental health through your whole body and whole self.

EMOTIONAL CHARACTERISTICS

The primary goal of this book is to help you develop a more loving and connected relationship with yourself. Part of that process is learning more about all the wonderful emotions within you. First, we'll start with the core emotions: happiness, sadness, fear, and anger.

Using the chart below, give each emotion a name, main features, and things that help you cope with or understand it, which we'll call "best friends."

EMOTION	NAME	MAIN FEATURES	BEST FRIENDS
(E.g., Anger)	(E.g., Frank)	(E.g., Short fuse, doesn't say much, barks sharply at others)	(E.g., Hitting the boxing bag, running, stream of consciousness writing, ten minutes of Tetris)
Happiness			
Sadness			
Fear			
Anger			

When you notice these emotions pop up in your life, remember their names, main features, and best friends. Then consider how this information can help you cope and navigate through these emotions.

KNOW YOUR SHIFTING MOODS

It is common to experience a sudden change in your emotions, which can subsequently derail your goals, motivation, or following your values. By tuning in with yourself and understanding the ways your emotions change, you can learn to navigate through them rather than be guided by them.

Think about when your mood changes or shifts. How do you know your mood is changing in the moment? For example, what goes on within you that tells you you're going from happy to sad?

_____

_____

_____

Name a few different scenarios where your emotions tend to suddenly shift (e.g., avoiding an accident, a sudden fight with someone).

_____

_____

_____

How would you explain this shift to others? Describe the physical feeling, different emotions, and overall experience.

_____

_____

_____

Negative and Positive Emotions

We often categorize negative and positive emotions in a "good" or "bad" binary. It's understandable, but instead of thinking of negative emotions as the antithesis of positive emotions, think of them as a collective of emotions working together as part of your complete human experience.

All this to say, mental health does not mean the absence of difficult feelings. Instead, mental health includes acknowledging and working through the various emotions and experiences that life throws at us.

It should be no surprise that most humans do what they can to avoid pain. So, it makes sense that we would also actively avoid difficult or painful emotions, especially if we weren't taught how to feel our way through emotions. The tricky part is that there's no possible way to avoid experiencing the breadth and depth of emotions, and avoiding them will only guarantee they come out sideways. Behaviors like road rage, hypochondria, and substance abuse are examples of emotions coming out in ways that work against you.

Although uncomfortable, the direct route through your emotions is the most beneficial and efficient way to process your experiences.

LISTENING TO YOUR EMOTIONS

Using the table below, fill in the characteristics of your emotions to better understand and relate to them in the future.

EMOTION	PHYSICAL SENSATION	ASSOCIATED MEMORY	TRAUMA/ VULNERABILITY
(E.g., Sadness)	*(E.g., Heavy head, pit in my stomach)*	*(E.g., Recent breakup)*	*(E.g., Abandonment trauma)*
Happiness			
Excitement			
Sadness			
Grief			
Anxiety			
Fear			
Surprise			
Anger			
Rage			

By having a fuller understanding of how these emotions show up in your life, you'll be able to identify when they occur, what they're connected to, and how to bring yourself down using another coping strategy.

SOAKING IN THE GOOD TIMES

While working on understanding yourself, it's necessary to look at parts of yourself that you're not proud of in order to accept yourself and enact change. However, positive psychology also encourages sitting with positive experiences. Some modalities call this "soaking."

Choose a positive memory, such as a graduation or achievement, and recount the experience through all of your available senses. The goal is to actively soak in a positive experience the next time you encounter one.

Positive memory:

_____

_____

What did the moment look like? Was it at night or during the day? Was it at your home or another location? Fill in the scene with the visuals.

_____

_____

What were the feelings on your skin? Was the weather cold or hot? What did your clothes feel like? Did you feel goose bumps?

_____

_____

What were some of the smells? Were you at home? Were you somewhere else? Write down the scents you smelled.

_____

_____

CONTINUED

How about taste? Were you eating or drinking anything? What did the air taste like?

_____

_____

What did you hear? Were you having a conversation? Was there deafening silence? Chirping birds? Fill in the scene.

_____

_____

SAMMY'S GRIEF STRUGGLE

Sammy was having a hard time with grief. After a decade of surgeries and various treatments, he had recently lost his mom to cancer. Sammy had a complicated relationship with his mom growing up, which made grieving trickier for him. In therapy, he found that he would be "shoulding all over himself," meaning he kept telling himself what he should or shouldn't be doing. When he cried while thinking about his mom, he would push the tears away and say, "I shouldn't be crying." If he felt sad when he woke up, he would say, "What's wrong with me? I should feel happy today."

After reading *Radical Acceptance* by Tara Brach, Sammy wondered what it would feel like to stop the "shoulding" and try to accept the feelings first. Over the next week, he would practice pausing and telling himself, "It's okay to grieve," whenever he felt a wave of sadness. He would breathe through the uncomfortable feelings that arose. "It's okay that I miss my mom," he would say as he cried. Additionally, he would try to divert himself when he started to judge his new sayings. If he caught himself being critical of his grieving process, he would try to say, "And now I'm judging myself for being kind to myself."

Over time, the compassionate self-observations allowed Sammy to continue to process his grief without the added feelings of shame and guilt impacting his healing.

Emotion Regulation

Regulating emotions involves tuning in to how you're feeling in the moment and knowing what you need to ground yourself. Put another way, you're asking yourself, "What am I feeling and how do I slow myself down?" Let's first go over an example of what this looks like.

Say your partner mentions they're going away with some friends this weekend. Suddenly, a wave of anxiety hits your gut. This experience is your "first reaction." Through self-awareness, you can name your reaction from a detached angle and think, *I'm feeling anxious at the idea of my partner leaving for a weekend because I will miss them and wish I could be with them.*

You don't act on that initial wave of anxiety, but use it to inform what you're reacting to and then decide on a response that works for you and your relationship. This process is known as the "second reaction." This is the reaction you give more energy to because it ideally involves self-awareness and squaring your values to your response.

A "second reaction" in this example can range anywhere from telling your partner, "Wow, I suddenly feel anxious, but that's separate from your time with friends. Have fun!" to "Eesh, that makes me anxious. Can we talk about this more before you go?" Of course, there are also many options between those ends of the spectrum.

Notice how none of the options included demanding your partner change their behavior. Although that can be a request later, it's essential that you start with naming and owning your emotional reactions.

Regulating emotions also means doing your best to give your mind and body what they need to make it easiest to regulate. When your emotional, psychological, and social needs are met, you are at your best ability to manage your emotions. I can have all this education and training in therapy, anxiety, and mindfulness, but it goes downhill fast if I am sleep deprived and hungry, for example.

Through my work, I've found that it's helpful to share what regulating emotions does **not** include, given the many misconceptions and stigma around being connected with your feelings. Emotional regulation is **not** ignoring your emotions by suppressing them. That's called dissociating, and although it might work in the short term, it's unfortunately a damaging long-term strategy. By tuning out or suppressing your emotions, you lose touch with your needs and boundaries over time. Suppressing your feelings has also been shown to increase physical illnesses and workplace stress.

EMOTIONAL OBSERVER

This is a mindfulness technique to help you create distance from your emotions. Pretend you are a researcher on an excursion to understand a newly discovered creature. You've heard about this being for years but never thought you'd get close to it. However, now you are going after this being to attempt to understand it fully.

This creature that you are following is your anxiety. Follow your anxiety as an observer and note what you see it doing. Try not to judge or manage it, but watch what happens and take note. Feel free to use what you learned in the Emotional Characteristics (page 19) and Listening to Your Emotions (page 22) activities to inform this exercise.

What behaviors are you seeing in your anxiety?

_____

_____

What happens when your anxiety gets more energy?

_____

_____

What happens when your anxiety peaks?

_____

_____

How does your anxiety naturally calm down?

_____

_____

What happens when you or someone else tries to control your anxiety?

_____

_____

INCREASE OVER TIME

Emotional regulation is not a skill you can turn on overnight, as you are likely noticing. One element of mindfulness in emotional regulation is slowly increasing your ability to sit with challenging emotions. If sitting with your eyes closed isn't comfortable for you, try doing these exercises while engaged in healthy movement.

When you experience an emotion like anxiety or sadness, instead of turning away from the emotion, try to turn toward it and mindfully examine how the feeling shows up.

1. Imagine there is a small box inside you, and in that box is that emotion. The emotion can only grow to the size of the box.

2. Now imagine the box slowly getting bigger but the emotion staying the same size.

3. Picture the emotion slowly filling in the excess space.

4. The box again slowly gets bigger, and the emotion stays the same size.

5. The emotion then fills that space.

It's okay if you need to do this exercise in multiple sessions. Reflect on the following prompts.

What did each step feel like?

_____

_____

_____

_____

Did you need a moment to pause or stop completely? If so, what told you that you needed to pause or stop?

_____

_____

_____

CONTINUED

What do you think would have happened if you didn't pause or stop?

_____

_____

_____

_____

What helped you expand your capacity to hold more of the emotion?

_____

_____

_____

_____

> *I am more than my emotions. Although my emotions work with me, they do not control me. I can have a healthy relationship with my feelings by being closer to them.*

What "Negative" Emotions Mean

Emotions can provide beneficial information to understand what's going on in your brain, life, and relationships. They are your body and mind's response to your inner life and environment. When experiencing an emotion that someone else has or feeling an emotion as a response to an event, you connect to the outside world. This can be a lovely way of navigating through your life. However, sometimes emotions take over or misfire due to chemical imbalances, negative self-esteem, or trauma.

Mental illness can occur when there is a neurochemical imbalance of gamma-aminobutyric acid, dopamine, or serotonin, resulting in difficulty regulating mood or thinking. These imbalances often result in diagnoses that include depression, schizophrenia, bipolar disorder, and mood disorders.

However, emotions are not only neurochemical phenomena. Instead, think of emotions as your body's "tuning fork" that can reverberate to frequencies around you. For example, if your boss is yelling at you, you will likely pick up on their emotion and react with anger or fear.

When feeling a "negative" emotion, try to understand the breadth of this emotion as part of your entire human experience, and not just as a "bad" emotion to be avoided. Challenging emotions can offer insight into unmet needs, value misalignment, or disrespected boundaries. Don't forget the power of reaching out for support when needed, too. You don't have to do this alone.

Anger and Irritability

Everyone experiences anger and irritability at some point. For some people, these reactive emotions seem to happen more often and can be disruptive. By understanding the various emotional states that contribute to anger and irritability, you can begin to address them more effectively.

Although you shouldn't minimize the importance and validity of anger or irritability, it is often a good idea to dig deeper into these emotions to find the other feelings playing a role in this experience. Irritability may seem minor, but it is often a warning signal for larger bouts of anger to come if left unattended. Tune into your anger and irritability and ask what else you are feeling. For example, are you also sad, anxious, or grieving? Is there an unmet need?

Sometimes anger results from injustice to yourself, someone you care about, or a larger community. This justifiable anger is a valid emotion of its own and is often joined with other emotions like sadness and despair. This is an example of where anger can be a driving force toward positive change.

You must clearly understand where the anger is coming from and what it's trying to address. Is it a result of a relational wound from childhood (e.g., your sibling was always the right one, and you were often sent to your room, so unfairness is a sticking point for you)? Is it a result of systemic injustice (e.g., unfair treatment of Black and Brown men in the criminal justice system)? Or is it from a partner that won't respect your boundaries despite repeated conversations (e.g., a partner that continues to cheat despite many conversations and apologies)? The point is to understand what is involved in your anger.

Anger, like anxiety, can start with an explosion so hot that it can feel impossible to find the ignition source. The goal is to slow yourself down and regulate your nervous system enough so you can think clearly alongside your anger.

CLOSER TO ANGER

Anger is often treated as a terrible thing that you should stay away from. Yet you can learn a lot about yourself by creating a nuanced relationship with anger through understanding the information within the emotion.

List three things that you know make you angry (e.g., being ignored, slow drivers, a critical boss)

1. _____
2. _____
3. _____

List three ways your body feels when you're angry.

1. _____
2. _____
3. _____

List three types of thoughts or phrases you have when you're angry (e.g., *What's wrong with people?*, calling people idiots while driving, etc.)

1. _____
2. _____
3. _____

Sometimes when you're angry, your thoughts and feelings may become rigid and convincing. What strategies can you use to approach the situation from a different angle? (e.g., asking what the underlying emotion may be to the anger, thinking about positive conversations with your boss and using that energy to address your concerns, etc.)

1. _____

2. _____

3. _____

4. _____

5. _____

6. _____

7. _____

8. _____

Who are three people you can reach out to when angry, or three activities to ground yourself?

1. _____

2. _____

3. _____

ABSOLUTE ANGER

Anger can have a convincing and intoxicating effect on you. The rising adrenaline, righteous indignation, and power felt through the emotion can often lead you into all-or-nothing thinking. Although it's not helpful to argue with your anger, it can be helpful to introduce curiosity and reflection to these moments to slow yourself down and ask, "What if I'm not 100 percent right?"

Using the table below, write down common all-or-nothing phrases you turn to while angry, then write a question or statement that helps with perspective-taking. Remember, you're not lying to yourself. You are taking an accurate account of the situation.

ABSOLUTE STATEMENT	QUESTION OR ACCURATE STATEMENT
(E.g., I'm such an idiot.)	*(E.g., I made a mistake.)*
(E.g., That's not fair.)	*(E.g., What's within my control to enact change?)*

Next time you find yourself in a moment of anger exclaiming one of these absolute statements, try to reflect on the question or accurate statement instead. This may be challenging while you are angry; if that's the case, then attempt to introduce this strategy as soon after the angry event as possible. By continuing to do this after each episode, you will close the gap over time and be able to check in with yourself while you are angry.

Anxiety and Nervousness

Anxiety is a feeling of unease, such as worry or fear, that can range from mild to intense. For some, anxiety can be so constant and overwhelming that it interferes with daily life. Although anxiety is sometimes seen as a negative emotion, it serves an essential purpose: keeping you safe. However, it can be debilitating when anxiety becomes too much to handle.

Sometimes a feeling of overwhelming anxiety is your body telling you something is meaningful to you. Do you get nervous before asking someone out on a date? Sweat buckets before presenting in front of your coworkers? Are you worried about a medical issue? These are all appropriate responses to important situations. However, it becomes an issue when the anxiety becomes so overwhelming that you either avoid the stressor altogether or you can't function.

Additionally, you've likely experienced some form of performance anxiety. Performance anxiety relates to an overwhelming sense of dread making it hard to focus and achieve your goals. This type of anxiety usually exists in three settings: sex, sports, and stage. Research has revealed that 30 to 60 percent of athletes experience performance anxiety, and 25 percent of men experience sexual performance anxiety.

In these moments, a person is stuck in a "fight, flight, freeze, or fawn" mode, or in the sympathetic nervous system, resulting in heightened anxiety and cognitive distortions. Mindfulness techniques can be helpful for these situations by helping you ground yourself, accept what is within your control, and focus on the present moment.

Through mindfulness techniques and committing to action within your control, you can increase your threshold for anxiety-provoking experiences. This is sometimes referred to as "pushing yourself to the edge of discomfort." The goal is to get you to the edge so you can test out the experience without being completely overwhelmed.

A CHALLENGING PERFORMANCE

You have likely experienced some form of performance anxiety. Right before a test, musical performance, or sex, you start to get racing thoughts expecting the worst. Fears of failure circle through your head, and it feels like you can't stop them.

Using the table below, consider different forms of performance anxiety and fill in the associated columns.

TYPE OF PERFORMANCE ANXIETY	MINDFULNESS TECHNIQUE	SAYING OF ACCEPTANCE	FOCUS ON OTHER FORMS OF SUCCESS
(E.g., sexual performance anxiety)	(E.g., deep breathing, focusing on other body parts, going slow)	(E.g., It's okay that this is happening. There are other ways to get pleasure and connect with my partner.)	(E.g., trying new activities, reminding self of incremental progress)

As a form of self-compassion, attempt to work in what you listed in the table when you are experiencing performance anxiety. Remember that this is a developmental process and it will take time to build the new habit, so it's important to be patient and kind to yourself.

SINK IN

This exercise comes from ACT (acceptance and commitment therapy), which encourages you to focus on one emotion at a time and accept it. You'll use tools learned from the Emotional Observer activity (page 26) for this exercise.

1. Sit comfortably and begin to take slow, deep breaths.

2. Mentally scan your body from the top of your head, throughout your body, and to your toes.

3. Identify any sensations that you are feeling.

4. After you slowly scan, identify where you most feel a particular emotion. For example, feeling a twist in your gut as a result of anxiety.

5. Continue by imagining yourself breathing *into* that sensation. Don't try to control it; just observe the feeling.

6. As you slowly breathe into the sensation, reflect on how the sensation may be changing.

7. Focus on the feeling while letting thoughts pass by. Continue to breathe. Give more definition to this sensation.

8. Now imagine you are allowing more space around this emotion and letting it take up more room if it wants. Continue to observe and not control it.

9. Place a hand on top of this sensation in a compassionate way. This hand is not to control but to hold and protect. When ready, you can lower your hand and open your eyes.

Use the space provided to write your reflections.

_____

_____

_____

_____

Shame and Guilt

Guilt and shame often get confused for each other, which is understandable because they're both part of a collection of social emotions. A social emotion relies on another person's thoughts, feelings, and actions about or toward you, which can be real or perceived. So, although depression or anxiety can occur independently, shame and guilt are often connected to a relationship with another person.

Within social emotions, we can differentiate between guilt and shame. Guilt is related to behavioral actions like things you do or don't do, whereas shame is related to who you are as a person. You can think of guilt as a remorseful act on its own, whereas shame is about the entirety of a person.

Furthermore, shame tells you you're worthless or no one cares about you. Shame tells you to hide. You may notice that when you feel ashamed, you likely pull away from seeing others or avoid eye contact. Combine this with the toxic masculine message that it's weak to talk about emotions or ask for help, and not only are you risking your mental health but also your life.

According to couples' therapist Terrence Real, "Men's willingness to downplay weakness and pain is so great that it has been named as a factor in their shorter life span. The ten years of difference in longevity between men and women turns out to have little to do with genes. Men wait longer to acknowledge that they are sick, take longer to get help, and once they get treatment do not comply with it as well as women do."

When you're overwhelmed with shame, ask yourself, "Who's opinion am I allowing to take over?" Since we sometimes need healthy levels of shame and guilt to follow our values and live in a community with others, it is helpful to explore these feelings and see if accountability is needed rather than completely banish them.

SHAME HANGOVER

You've been there. It's the day after a party or a big meeting, and you're standing in front of the mirror kicking yourself at that one thing you said or didn't say. Some refer to this as the "shame hangover," or as therapists call it, "rumination." Although this is a common experience for many people, it is helpful to know when it's happening and what to do.

Using the table below, write down common shame hangover thoughts you have in the first column, like, "I was stupid," or "Did I say something offensive?" Then fill in the remaining rows to begin unpacking the shame.

SHAME HANGOVER THOUGHT	CORE EMOTION	WHAT HAPPENED? ONLY LIST OBSERVABLE FACTS	WHAT IS MY PRIMARY CONCERN?	COMPASSIONATE REFLECTIONS	DID I CHECK IN?
(E.g., I was so stupid last night.)	(E.g., Humiliation)	(E.g., I made a joke, and no one laughed)	(E.g., Rejection)	(E.g., Remind self of times people laughed at my jokes)	(E.g., No)

Take some time and reflect on whether there are any themes or patterns in your shame hangovers, and use this as information to further understand areas of life that deserve attention and compassion.

INCREASING SELF-COMPASSION

Shame is fraught with self-criticism. It's a function of either punishing yourself or shutting yourself down. Pretty rough, right? One of the needed elements in healing from shame is self-compassion. However, many guys feel embarrassed by some self-compassionate statements. I encourage you to challenge any desire to feel cool or stoic over your need for mental health, but I also strongly believe in finding something that works for you.

Review and consider using some of these common self-compassion statements. Feel free to revise the statements in your own words in the space provided, or to write your own.

I can make mistakes while learning.

_____

Forgiving myself is part of progress.

_____

I accept the best and worst parts of myself.

_____

I accept and love my flaws.

_____

I am a patient and kind person.

_____

I am strong and beautiful as I am.

_____

Melancholy and Sadness

Some people think that melancholy and sadness are negative emotions that should be avoided at all costs. However, allowing yourself to fully experience these emotions can be a great source of wisdom and compassion.

Melancholy and sadness are not the opposite of happiness and joy, and they add to the emotional experiences of life. Sometimes they are connected to a longing for unmet needs, disappointment related to crossed boundaries, or missing someone. By tuning into the feeling's root, you gain information on your values, who you are as a person, and potentially find the necessary steps toward change. This process differs from that of those with severe mental illness, where depression has consumed the person.

Lastly, some men enter a state of depression after a physical injury or impairment to their ability to work or engage in their favorite hobby. When this occurs, it is a form of mourning the aspects of self-identity and sense of self that have changed. By taking time to honor this difference, you can process through the grief leading to acceptance and changing what's within your control.

CHECKING SADNESS

Sometimes sadness can deceptively consume your entire self by sneaking up on you and taking up space. For many men, anger is a common symptom of depression or sadness. Others experience sadness through slow movements or a lack of motivation. Knowing how sadness impacts you enables you to track it early on and get help before it becomes overwhelming.

Review the list below and check the signs of sadness that most stand out to you.

☐ Anger

☐ Low motivation

☐ Sleeping less

☐ Sleeping a lot

☐ Difficulty staying asleep

☐ Difficulty sitting still

☐ Crying spells

☐ Hypochondria

☐ Feeling empty

☐ Eating more or less than usual

☐ Low interest in activities you once enjoyed

☐ Difficulty holding attention

☐ Avoiding social events

☐ Avoiding your partner or family

☐ Increased time with videos or video games

☐ Mood swings

☐ Thoughts of suicide

☐ Planning suicide

☐ Hopelessness

☐ Guilt

☐ Weight gain

☐ Weight loss

When you know your signs of sadness, you can keep an eye on them when one or more shows up. These will be parts of your early warning system to acknowledge when you need to tend to your mental health.

CHATTING WITH SADNESS

Sadness can often feel like that unwanted visitor overstaying their welcome. Perhaps you try not to open the door when it arrives or attempt to ignore it so it just leaves on its own. However, as you learn from mindfulness and ACT, the most efficient approach is to meet your emotions head-on and accept them for what they are.

Using information from the Emotional Characteristics (page 19) and Listening to Your Emotions (page 22) exercises, have a chat with your sadness. Imagine you're sitting down across from sadness for an interview. Don't try to intimidate or appease your guest; instead, just learn more. You'll learn about healthy communication later, but in the meantime, use your best judgment to approach your sadness with curiosity and empathy.

What questions do you have about your sadness?

_____

_____

_____

_____

What do you think your sadness would say to you?

_____

_____

_____

_____

What questions would your sadness have for you?

_____

_____

_____

_____

CONTINUED

What's something you'd like to say to your sadness?

_____

_____

_____

_____

MOHAMMED'S DIFFICULT DATE

Mohammed felt a wave of both fear and excitement while getting ready for his date. He had been on several dates in the last few months, yet none of them were a match. However, he felt like tonight's date was a perfect fit for him. "I really hope this works out," he told himself while noticing he was even fantasizing about future dates and vacations with her.

However, the more he sat in the thought *I really hope this works out*, the more pressure he felt to do well on the date. The anxiety was so intense that he started to feel like he had no other choice but to get it right. He even convinced himself that tonight was his last chance for love. This anxiety led him to consider all the ways he could embarrass himself in front of his date. "What if I get too drunk? Spill food on my shirt? Have nothing to talk about? What if I can't get hard?"

With each question, his heart raced faster. Thankfully, he remembered his workbook from his dating coach and went through grounding exercises for his dating anxiety. Mohammed recognized that he was jumping to conclusions and setting unrealistic expectations for a first date. He felt an enormous sense of relief after reminding himself that he just needed to show up and he could figure out the rest later down the line. By focusing on the present moment, he could slow himself down and reduce the spiraling anxious thoughts.

Expressing How You Feel

You have learned that part of your emotions' role is facilitating communication with others in your life. However, you can't always clearly communicate just through your feelings. You also need to learn how to clearly express to others your emotional experiences. But how can you clearly express your feelings when you're used to funneling them out?

You've probably made many attempts to express your emotions in your life. Perhaps you experienced being shut down or ridiculed for expressing your emotions. Typically, when someone shuts down a man's emotional expression, it is likely because of one or more of the following reasons:

1. There's a gendered expectation for boys or men to be unexpressive.

2. The other person does not know how to offer support, so they push away.

3. The individual expressing their emotion has a history of sharing their emotions violently and/or without boundaries for themselves or others.

How has your view of masculinity influenced how you express your feelings? Many men find expressing their emotions a threat to their masculinity. One study found that men who scored high in conforming to a strong sense of masculinity were rated lower in terms of emotional vulnerability. Expressing your feelings can be seen as going against masculine values, but the same study showed that gender norms are slowly evolving to be less fear-based and more empowerment-based.

When expressing your feelings, it is important to be informed by your emotions but not consumed by them. Sharing your emotions with someone else requires you to be vulnerable, grounded, and self-aware. Do you need these skills before starting? Nope. You can develop them as you go, but do your best to make them a priority in your healing journey. Otherwise, you may force your partner into a position of either emotionally caring for you on demand, or potentially coming across as neglectful if they set boundaries. This often pushes people away and may add to a narrative that "no one cares about me."

Although you deserve social support in life, you also have to do the work to help others help yourself. Throughout the workbook, you will continue to build your emotional regulation, cognitive processing, and social skills to provide the necessary foundation for others to support you.

LABELING YOUR FEELINGS

Before you express your feelings, you'll first need to learn how to identify and label them. By being able to label your feelings, you can then identify what you need for coping or support.

Using the table below, fill in the different sensations you experience related to each emotion. This will help you in the future to label the emotions based on the indicators you list below. It's okay if you aren't able to answer right away. This exercise is designed to help you identify your emotional experience over time.

EMOTION	PHYSICAL SENSATION	ASSOCIATED THOUGHTS	IMPACT	COPING STRATEGIES
(Ex., Anger)	*(Heat in chest, balling up fists)*	*(I go blank, but I feel very focused)*	*(My heart rate goes up; my coworkers seem worried)*	*(Deep breathing)*
Anger				
Anxiety				
Sadness				
Shame				

Through the information you filled in above, you can now work to spot these emotions when they are showing up, and follow your coping strategies associated with the emotion.

SHAME GAME

This isn't a game to play when you're feeling great, but it is a quick and simple exercise to help accurately reframe the tricky social emotions you experience.

Using a simple formula, differentiate the actions you have committed from who you are as a person: "Just because I did X, does not mean that I *am* Y."

Let's say you were overwhelmed with many projects and were late for a work deadline. Taken over by shame, you feel like you're the worst employee and will be fired soon. The formula for this example would be, "Just because I missed the deadline does not mean that I am a bad employee."

Try some others using the templates provided below:

"Just because I _____,

does not mean that I *am*_____."

"Just because I _____,

does not mean that I *am*_____."

"Just because I _____,

does not mean that I *am*_____."

Next time you feel shame or embarrassment, try to reframe the situation into this formula to help you get perspective on the specific issue rather than a generally negative view of yourself.

Developing Resiliency

Every day, you experience different types of stress in your life. It could be from work, family, or health problems. Although some stress is common, chronic and unmanaged stress can negatively affect your mental and physical health. One way to protect yourself from the harmful effects of stress is to develop resilience: the ability to adapt and cope with difficult situations. There are many things you can do to build resilience.

Resiliency, like mental health, includes attuning to your physical, emotional, and social needs. Other factors include communication skills, gratitude, compassion, mindfulness, and empathy. Rick Hanson, a psychologist at UC Berkeley who focuses on resiliency, discusses the importance of "grit" in resilience. Grit is the combination of passion and perseverance, or the ability to push through adversity because a value or purpose drives you. This can include challenging life events such as schooling, boot camp, medical hardships, and (for some guys) emotionally challenging conversations with their partners. What are some parts of your life where you display grit?

It's essential to differentiate resilience from "taking everything on." Resiliency doesn't mean being able to handle anything and everything. Resiliency includes setting and maintaining boundaries and knowing your capacity for which projects you agree to. This will help manage the number of responsibilities in your life. By knowing what you can do, learning how long projects will take, and being able to say yes or no to them, you maintain your system in a way that doesn't overwhelm you with stress. This way, you are not overextending yourself, dropping the ball on responsibilities that need more attention, and then feeling poorly about yourself.

Some men have difficulty with resiliency for various reasons, not including circumstances involving severe mental illness or systemic issues outside their control. For example, capitalist influences tell you that your worthiness relies on your ability to work and produce; patriarchy tells you to push your feelings down and not express them; and both prioritize individualism over collectivism, leaving many men feeling isolated and alone.

Ideally, through challenging the pressures we have received, you can inspect them and decide for yourself which values you want to follow. Cultivating your own sense of resiliency can lead to a greater understanding of self, increased longevity, lower depression, and overall life satisfaction.

DAY BY DAY

Mental health includes experiencing the full range of the emotional spectrum. However, even with mental health, you will experience "bad days." What's important is to recognize and accept the natural ebb and flow of our moods.

Over the next week, use the calendar below to track your emotions three times a day and reflect on what you learn about yourself.

Day	Morning (E.g., feeling anxiety in the morning)	Midday (E.g., feeling quiet and flat)	Evening (E.g., feeling lonely)
MONDAY			
TUESDAY			
WEDNESDAY			
THURSDAY			
FRIDAY			
SATURDAY			
SUNDAY			

TICK-TOCK

One aspect of accessing emotions includes knowing the sensations and experience of shifting moods. Like a pendulum, you will naturally experience a swinging of emotions, so understanding the sensations and thoughts associated with the swinging back and forth can help you ground yourself.

1. Think of a time when you felt sad or down. Imagine it and feel it in your body.

2. Now think of a time when you felt happy or up. Imagine that and feel it in your body.

3. Imagine feeling down again.

4. Now imagine feeling up again.

5. Continue this process three times.

What does it feel like to go from feeling down to up? How about from feeling up to down? What thoughts, emotions, and bodily sensations are associated with this emotional transition?

_____

_____

_____

_____

> *Developing a healthy relationship is not an obligation. I choose to work on myself. Understanding who I am and how I relate to the world around me contributes to my life satisfaction.*

Chapter Reflection

Well done! You made it to the end of this emotional chapter. Sure, it's not climbing Mount Kilimanjaro, but it's enough of an achievement to warrant reflection and gratitude. In this chapter, you learned about how emotions like anger, anxiety, and shame can impact you, as well as ways to navigate through these experiences. Please take a moment to consider how you can apply some of the tenets and exercises of this chapter to your day-to-day life. As you sit with this book, take deep breaths, and recall which aspects stood out most. Get curious about why these portions of the text resonated with you. How will you approach these areas of your life differently now?

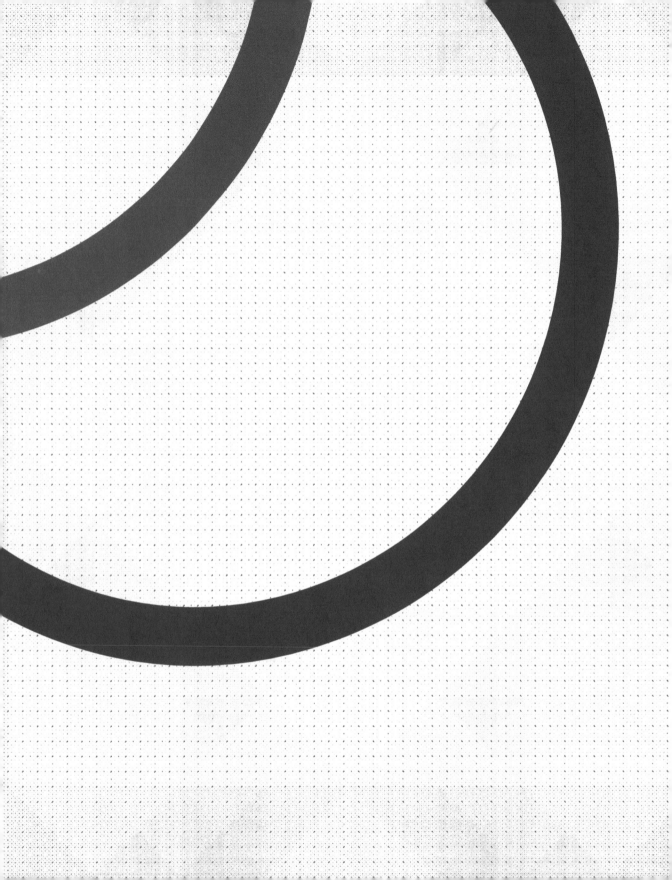

CHAPTER THREE

PSYCHOLOGICAL MENTAL HEALTH

> *I decide what masculinity means to me.*
> *No one else can define my gender or its*
> *expression in my life. I can take*
> *inspiration from whomever I want.*

How You Think

Many men I've worked with hold an expectation of themselves to always be strong and decisive. This stance was modeled to them by men they idolized while growing up, who took pride in their ability to make quick decisions and never show weakness. But what are the benefits to men who hold themselves to this extreme? In this chapter, you'll explore how men can benefit from thinking more deliberately and openly about their thoughts and feelings, rather than shoving them away. You'll also look at how traditional ideas about masculinity can hold us back from achieving our full potential. It's time to start thinking differently.

Most men are socialized to address concerns with a "fix-it" attitude. This approach isn't wrong on its own, but can be a challenge when some issues can't be solved immediately. Those issues, such as processing grief, deserve time and compassion through emotional connection rather than only giving tactical support.

Social conditioning tells everyone to fix, cure, and produce or else we risk our value in society. Even more so, social pressure puts many men in a position of asserting control or dominance, which then frames thinking, strategy, and relationships as a power struggle. This struggle adds competition or risk to thinking and relating. Therefore, it becomes more important to be correct rather than understand or connect. Of course, there are exceptions to the rule, but take a moment and consider how this can play out in your thinking.

During your time with this workbook, consider how you approach thinking from a "fix-it" or "dominator" model and decide when those models are appropriate, and which other approaches can work as a more effective strategy.

PAUL'S PROGRAMMER PREDICAMENT

Paul has been a programmer since he got his first computer when he was twelve years old. His mind was naturally drawn toward problem-solving, and he felt joy when he fixed an issue in rapid time. But unfortunately, while this skill worked wonderfully for his career, it was a losing strategy for connection in his romantic relationship.

Time and time again, he would be met with frustration and exasperation from his partner when she came to him about her issues and concerns. She told him that even though she knew he was coming from a good place, his problem-solving felt like he wasn't listening to her and that he was either minimizing her issues or pushing her away. For Paul, his experience was that he *was* listening intently while hearing her pain, and to him, the next logical step was to help her alleviate the pain.

Paul shared this with her again, which was helpful as a reminder about his intentions. However, his partner shared that the impact of how he shared this advice wasn't a winning strategy for feeling closer together. If anything, she shared, it felt like he was talking down to her.

Through acceptance and compassion, Paul could hear that his partner wasn't putting him down or telling him he was wrong. Paul realized it wasn't about right and wrong but more about him and his partner learning about and accepting each other. As a result, Paul agreed to ask his partner before giving advice, which gave them the option to work together and support each other.

Science of Your Brain

Research in neuroplasticity has given the scientific community a great deal of understanding about how the brain works, adapts, and learns. However, there's so much more to discover. Neuroplasticity refers to the changes in the nervous system and brain due to lived experiences. Plasticity, in this case, means that it is moveable and adaptable. Therefore, the neurons in your brain are trainable through various exercises and interventions. Although your brain rapidly grows during childhood, adolescence, and early adulthood, it continues to develop throughout your life, allowing you to create new and more adaptive neural pathways.

However, just as you can adapt to positive forms of change, you can also develop neural pathways that establish a view of the world that can work against you. Negativity bias is a natural human tendency to add more weight to negative experiences than positive ones. You may resonate with the idea that you can give a speech to a hundred people where ninety-nine of them are thrilled with what you're saying, but you base how the talk went on the one yawning guy who rolled his eyes the whole time. From an evolutionary perspective, it makes sense that you would seek information on threats to safety or belonging. However, this can often show up in ways that undermine your relationship with yourself and others.

Thankfully, there are ways to combat negativity bias. First, by acknowledging the entirety of the facts in front of you, you can get an accurate assessment of the situation. This way, you're not lying to yourself, but you are reminding yourself of the truth that ninety-nine people loved your talk. More on that will be covered later. The important part is to know that your brain and values can still change and adapt to your environment no matter how old you are.

CHALLENGING NEGATIVITY BIAS

Using the table below, write out significant themes for you and then follow the rows to work through them. An "accepting statement" is one that simply states the facts of what you are going through without judging or attempting to change your reality. A "changing behavior" is an action that you are committed to doing in order to work against negativity bias. Recognizing these themes will help you manage your bias.

THEME OF BIAS	SPECIFIC EXAMPLE	ACCEPTING STATEMENT	CHANGING BEHAVIOR
(E.g., Loneliness)	*(E.g., Feeling despair while dating)*	*(E.g., Yes, I'm overwhelmed by dating. But it helps me learn what I'm looking for in a partner.)*	*(E.g., Use what I learned from dating to refine my search for a partner)*

The next time you notice a negativity bias show up, follow your own accepting statement and changing behavior to help cope and adjust.

RETRAINING YOUR BRAIN
THROUGH BREATHING

In this exercise, you'll learn about body scan meditation as a form of rest and restoration for your mind and body.

1. Find a comfortable place to lie down and close your eyes.

2. Begin to focus on your breathing, without controlling it. Notice the natural pacing.

3. Once you've established your breathing, notice how your body feels overall. Where does it feel warm? What muscles are you tensing? Is there any pain or discomfort?

4. Begin to scan your body, starting at your toes mentally. Notice how your feet and legs feel.

5. Scan your pelvis and buttocks. Continue to breathe. What sensations are you feeling?

6. Notice your torso, including your gut, chest, and shoulders. What sensations do you feel?

7. Slowly scan the back of your head, up to your scalp, and then slowly down your face.

This practice may not seem like much, but if kept up, consistent meditation can improve neuroplasticity and reduce cognitive decline.

Trauma Responses and Mental Health

It is common for people who have experienced a traumatic event to feel like they are living in a different world. Trauma can impact how they view themselves and the world around them. It is important to understand how trauma can affect someone so that you can provide the support they need. Trauma can change how people see themselves, their relationships, and their world. This can be very challenging to deal with, but there are ways to get help. If you are struggling after experiencing a traumatic event, please reach out for help. You are not alone, and you can find resources in the back of this book to assist you.

Your brain and nervous system store memories of traumatic or threatening events as a protective measure. This is incredibly useful for survival. However, post-traumatic stress disorder (PTSD) can cause your trauma response to activate at unneeded times, often impacting your mood, sense of safety, and relationships.

Everyone has a "window of tolerance," which is the space between hyperarousal and hypoarousal. You can stay in your window of tolerance by knowing what helps your emotional regulation. However, stress and trauma will impact how spacious your window of tolerance can remain. For example, your tolerance for frustration and further stress is understandably minimal if you are already overwhelmed and stressed. So, if you experience constant work-related stress, an abusive relationship, or any recurring trauma, your mood and ability to cope are impacted.

Hyperarousal: anxiety, fight or flight, rage, out of control, overwhelmed; hyperaware of your surroundings

Window of Tolerance: grounded and able to withstand the ups and downs of daily life

Hypoarousal: foggy headed, dissociated, zoned out, spacey; minimally aware of your surroundings

---

This is far from an exhaustive explanation of what happens with trauma and mental health, but merely a quick overview. Please refer to the Resources and References sections (pages 123 and 125) for further reading and understanding of trauma and mental health.

Depression and Depressive States

When feeling down, most people might say they are feeling depressed. However, clinical depression is a different story. Although many factors can lead to a depressive state that may only last for a short time, clinical depression is a severe mental health condition that requires treatment. Therefore, knowing the difference between the two is essential in getting the help you need.

A depressive state is often depression related to a life event or environmental stressor. This form of depression can be related to grief, losing a job, medical issues, loneliness, breakups/divorce, and so on. The length of time one is in this state largely depends on situational and cultural factors.

Clinical depression is a mood disorder associated with prolonged periods (longer than six months) where depressive symptoms overwhelm the person and severely impact daily functioning. This type of depression is related to a neurochemical imbalance and is sometimes resistant to formal modes of treatment. However, in some cases, alternative treatment methods like psychedelic-assisted therapy have been shown to improve the mood of severely depressed patients.

Some of the exercises in the workbook address depression, because it's not only essential to know how to cope with depression but also helpful to know what it looks like. What are the warning signs of depression?

- Feeling "empty," "numb," or "flat"
- Anger
- Difficulty staying still
- Low energy
- Not finding joy in things you used to enjoy doing

- Sleeping too much or too little
- Severely changed appetite
- Isolating from others
- Suicidal thoughts

Untreated depression has taken the lives of so many men. The best things to do for depression are to be kind to yourself, seek support from trusted people and trained professionals, and attempt to make movements every day toward improving your mental health, no matter how small they may seem. These can be literal movements like exercise or yoga, or they can be completing tasks pertinent to your well-being.

YOUR DEPRESSIVE CHECKLIST

When you are feeling low and are concerned that you're showing signs of depression, use this checklist to see if you match some of the criteria. Throughout the week, check all the ones that apply to you.

MONDAY	☐ Little interest or joy in doing things ☐ Feeling down, depressed, or hopeless ☐ Trouble falling or staying asleep, or sleeping too much ☐ Poor appetite, overeating, or considerable weight changes ☐ Feeling bad about yourself ☐ Difficulty concentrating on things or making decisions ☐ Thoughts that you would be better off dead or hurting yourself
TUESDAY	☐ Little interest or joy in doing things ☐ Feeling down, depressed, or hopeless ☐ Trouble falling or staying asleep, or sleeping too much ☐ Poor appetite, overeating, or considerable weight changes ☐ Feeling bad about yourself ☐ Difficulty concentrating on things or making decisions ☐ Thoughts that you would be better off dead or hurting yourself

WEDNESDAY	☐ Little interest or joy in doing things ☐ Feeling down, depressed, or hopeless ☐ Trouble falling or staying asleep, or sleeping too much ☐ Poor appetite, overeating, or considerable weight changes ☐ Feeling bad about yourself ☐ Difficulty concentrating on things or making decisions ☐ Thoughts that you would be better off dead or hurting yourself
THURSDAY	☐ Little interest or joy in doing things ☐ Feeling down, depressed, or hopeless ☐ Trouble falling or staying asleep, or sleeping too much ☐ Poor appetite, overeating, or considerable weight changes ☐ Feeling bad about yourself ☐ Difficulty concentrating on things or making decisions ☐ Thoughts that you would be better off dead or hurting yourself
FRIDAY	☐ Little interest or joy in doing things ☐ Feeling down, depressed, or hopeless ☐ Trouble falling or staying asleep, or sleeping too much ☐ Poor appetite, overeating, or considerable weight changes ☐ Feeling bad about yourself ☐ Difficulty concentrating on things or making decisions ☐ Thoughts that you would be better off dead or hurting yourself

CONTINUED

SATURDAY	☐ Little interest or joy in doing things ☐ Feeling down, depressed, or hopeless ☐ Trouble falling or staying asleep, or sleeping too much ☐ Poor appetite, overeating, or considerable weight changes ☐ Feeling bad about yourself ☐ Difficulty concentrating on things or making decisions ☐ Thoughts that you would be better off dead or hurting yourself
SUNDAY	☐ Little interest or joy in doing things ☐ Feeling down, depressed, or hopeless ☐ Trouble falling or staying asleep, or sleeping too much ☐ Poor appetite, overeating, or considerable weight changes ☐ Feeling bad about yourself ☐ Difficulty concentrating on things or making decisions ☐ Thoughts that you would be better off dead or hurting yourself

If you selected two or more of these symptoms for two or more days within a week, I encourage you to schedule a check-in with a doctor or therapist. If that isn't possible right now, please refer to the Resources list at the end of this book (page 123) for other affordable options.

VALUES ALIGNER

Many refer to their values as their north star, or guiding light. Your values are your guiding principles to help you understand yourself and your relationships, and to assist you in making decisions. Making choices through the framework of your values can greatly improve your mental health because you are acting in ways that help you like yourself.

Below is a lengthy but not exhaustive list of values. Please check the ones that resonate with you the most. There is space at the end to write in your own.

☐ Altruism	☐ Integrity
☐ Appreciation	☐ Kindness
☐ Attentiveness	☐ Loyalty
☐ Compassion	☐ Self-reliance
☐ Courage	☐ Selflessness
☐ Dependability	☐ Spirituality
☐ Determination	☐ Tolerance
☐ Empathy	☐ Toughness
☐ Equanimity	☐ Trustworthiness
☐ Generosity	☐ _____
☐ Gratitude	☐ _____
☐ Honesty	☐ _____
☐ Humility	

CONTINUED

Out of the ones you've chosen, write down two or three that you consider your core values. These will be some of your main guiding principles.

_____

_____

_____

Addictions and Compulsive Behaviors

The most challenging part about addictions is that they work well in meeting their goal . . . at least in the short term. A person engages in addictive or compulsive behavior to soothe some emotion or craving, and the nature of what they're seeking makes it so that the "thing" works quickly to comfort them. For example, cigarettes, alcohol, cocaine, gambling, and sex can give an immediate reward and flood the brain with enough neurochemicals to act like a warm hug or an exciting distraction. Even seemingly harmless things like social media, shopping, and food can develop into compulsive and destructive behaviors.

So, we first must acknowledge that there's a reason why someone has an addiction or compulsive behavior. Despite the costs associated with the addiction or behavior, there are still valid reasons why people engage in them, and to ignore that fact would just be putting a bandage over the issue. As an example of under-lying problems, Carl Hart, a leading neuroscientist researcher on addictions, wrote, "a great deal of pathological drug use is driven by unmet social needs, by being alienated and having difficulty connecting with others."

That's why when you think about addiction for yourself or someone else, it's vital to be non-shaming and compassionate while also realistic about how the addiction or compulsions impact your life. Substance misuse, abuse, and some compulsive behaviors can actively interfere with your mental health. The interference is related to the effects on your neurochemistry, like dopamine and adrenaline, and your ability to use different coping skills.

There are a tremendous number of books and research on addiction and mental health, and if this is something you are struggling with, there are many ways to receive support. Please consult the Resources section at the back of the book (page 123) for guidance and options.

DRIVING WITH YOUR THOUGHTS

Imagine that you are driving a bus, and your passengers are your thoughts. You are riding with your passengers, but they are not the ones directing you. During the drive, some of your passengers are encouraging and polite while others call you nasty names and put you down.

You can choose how you want to engage with and react to these passengers. For example, while working on your breathing, you can focus on the road even while some passengers are trying to distract you with verbal attacks.

Your passengers may even try to direct you down roads that lead to choices that work against your larger goals and values. Consider how you want to respond to the passengers' demands within this thought exercise.

This exercise can be a helpful metaphor to carry with you as a reminder that you can have distance from your thoughts, and even though they may be with you at all times, you can choose how to interact with them.

KNOWING YOUR "WHY"

Addressing addiction or compulsive behaviors is a challenging but worthy effort. Understanding what is underneath your relationship to the addiction or compulsion can help support your process. Consider doing this exercise even if you don't believe you have a challenging relationship with substances or any compulsions. Your reflections may illuminate some areas to pay closer attention to.

In the space below, write down two or three addictive or compulsive behaviors you want to change or observe more directly.

_____

_____

_____

Write down the reasons you think you turn toward those behaviors. Bonus points if you can include what you are avoiding by seeking these behaviors out.

(**Example:** *I start to drink on Fridays to blow off some steam because of work stress. I think it helps me forget about how little I care about my job, but it doesn't change my career in the long run.*)

_____

_____

_____

_____

> *Just because I made a mistake does not mean I am doomed to fail the entire process. On the contrary, mistakes are necessary for learning and do not define who I am.*

How Stress Affects the Brain

You know that stress isn't good for you. You feel it in your muscles, your mind, and sometimes even in your physical appearance. Studies have shown that chronic stress can lead to changes in your brain structure and functioning, which can cause problems with cognitive performance, memory, and emotional well-being.

In a stressful situation, your brain registers the event as a threat that signals your mind and body to prepare to survive. This shift into the sympathetic nervous system results in a rush of cortisol and adrenaline through your body, which causes increased heart rate, blood rushing to your primary organs, rapid breathing, and reduced digestion. This is an entirely necessary reaction to threats to your survival. However, you may likely experience heightened stress unrelated to survival. What happens to the brain when stress related to work, relationships, discrimination, or trauma continues throughout your life?

With the consistent increase in adrenaline and cortisol levels, you can be more susceptible to cognitive impairments like memory loss, Alzheimer's disease, or dementia. One part of the brain related to stress management is the hippocampus, which is responsible for memory and learning. One study showed that stress impacts the hippocampus and shrinks this part of your brain, so repeated stress or trauma can significantly impact your cognitive functioning. Other studies have shown that cortisol and adrenaline can increase the chances of severe mental health issues in those predisposed to these illnesses due to genetics or environmental factors.

You may already be able to see how your brain's reaction to stress can affect your relationships with others. When you are in a fight, flight, freeze, or fawn mode, you may react to those around you as threats. Sadly, the people in your life will end up hurt when you take out your stress on them. What can happen in these situations is that others in your life create boundaries from you to help buffer the impact of your stress. Their reaction can lead you to take that information as further "proof" that others won't support you. In fact, repeated stress can increase your chances of engaging in negativity bias and learned helplessness. So, the goal is to learn how to manage stress in your life and develop boundaries to reduce the controllable stress. Does this mean that if stress hurts your relationships, you're not trying hard enough? Nope. It's important to identify and accept what is actually within your control to create any number of boundaries to lower the stress in your life.

BELLY BOX BREATHING

Stress offers a one-two punch against your mental health. It impacts both your thoughts and your nervous system. This exercise works to soothe both by working on your breathing and giving your mind something to focus on.

1. Sit or lie in a comfortable position.

2. Close your eyes or softly gaze in front of you.

3. Now breathe in for 4 seconds while expanding your belly slowly. Hold that breath for 4 seconds.

4. Then breathe out for 4 seconds and bring your belly in. Once again, hold your breath for 4 seconds.

5. Repeat this four times.

6. Continue to breathe and hold while expanding and contracting your belly, but begin to imagine a line drawing up on the next breath in.

7. Then imagine the line turning right while you hold your breath.

8. The line then drops down as you breathe out for 4 seconds.

9. Finally, the line turns left and completes the box while you hold your breath.

10. Repeat this box breathing process four more times.

Reflect on how you feel after this breathing exercise. How does your body feel? What are your thoughts like? What sensations or memories are coming up?

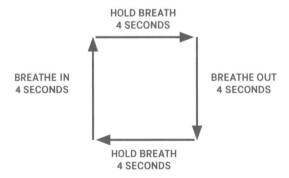

FINDING JOY

Accessing positive memories or acknowledging your own areas of confidence can be an excellent addition to your resiliency tool kit. Using the space below, list out positive memories and accomplishments that you want to remember often.

Happy memories (e.g., cooking a hot meal and enjoying it on a cold day):

_____

_____

_____

_____

Accomplishments (e.g., consistently working out for six months, graduating college, etc.):

_____

_____

_____

_____

Consider revisiting these lists, and even adding to them, when you find yourself struggling and need to find your joy.

Handling Stress

As discussed in the resiliency section in chapter 2 (page 45), the goal of handling stress isn't to simply and brutally take whatever is thrown at you. Instead, a significant component of handling stress is knowing your capacity and being able to set boundaries regarding what's within your control. This way, you can preserve your energy and attention to handle existing stress without piling more in the background.

For men, stress typically comes in three forms: pressure to perform, pressure to provide, and struggle to meet unrealistic expectations. With all three stress areas, one way to work through it is to know how much you can take on and how to push away the rest. Figuring out your capacity can take a while, but it's worth the effort to check in with yourself and acknowledge how much is on your plate. By recognizing your current external stressors (e.g., work, medical issues, parenting, etc.) you can gauge how much you can take on.

Of course, being able to control such external pressures is often easier said than done. However, identifying what you have within your control can be grounding and empowering.

Beyond establishing boundaries, learning coping skills that work for you is essential in handling stress. There's no one right way to engage in coping skills. What's important is to find the ones that address your concerns in a way you can process. Examples include:

- Exercise/sports
- Individual/group therapy
- Yoga

- Meditation
- Hobbies
- Creative arts

As you can see, there's not one particular way to process stress. One person may benefit from strenuous exercise, whereas another benefits from meditation.

Please note: Don't hold yourself back from doing certain activities or hobbies because it may be outside of gender norms. This is for you. Your life is for you, and so is your comfort. Whether your idea of dealing with stress involves jiujitsu or pole dancing, crochet or woodworking, it makes no difference. All that matters is that you get to center yourself. Don't let others' naive judgments hold you back from grounding yourself.

STRESS SAFETY SACK

Remember, stress impacts your *entire* system: your mind, body, nervous system, and relationships. Of course, the paradox is that it's tough to get the motivation or time for self-care when you need it the most. Figuring out what you need in your tool kit, or safety sack, ahead of time can help take away some of the barriers to grounding yourself when you're stressed. Because stress impacts many aspects of your life, let's break down your self-care to address each domain. Some activities may apply to many areas. If so, that's even better!

Identify activities in the following areas that will help reduce stress:

Physical (e.g., yoga, hiking, basketball, massage):

_____

_____

_____

_____

Senses (e.g., listening to music, lighting candles, cooking, taking a bath):

_____

_____

_____

_____

Emotional (e.g., journaling, letting yourself cry, calling a friend):

_____

_____

_____

_____

CONTINUED

STRESS SAFETY SACK CONTINUED

Creative (e.g., painting, woodworking, karaoke):

_____

_____

_____

_____

Social (e.g., team sports, board games, casual cookout):

_____

_____

_____

_____

Cognitive (e.g., puzzles, Tetris, coding challenge):

_____

_____

_____

_____

Spiritual (e.g., meditation; prayer; visiting a temple, mosque, or church):

_____

_____

_____

_____

LABEL AND SORT

Labeling your thoughts can be a useful practice in getting distance from them. By doing so, you can note them, understand their role, and then let them move on.

Take some time out of your day to watch your thoughts float by and label them as accurately as possible. Then see how specific you can get in your description over time. Begin by labeling the core emotion behind the thought, like joy, anxiety, sadness, shame, etc. Then try associating the thought with a value, need, boundary, memory, or trauma. In other words, what else is connected to this thought?

Use the space provided to write down notes on this exercise.

Thought:

_____

_____

_____

_____

Core emotion:

_____

_____

_____

_____

Connections to the thought (value, need, boundary, memory, trauma, etc.):

_____

_____

_____

_____

Cultivating Gratitude

What do you imagine when you think about "cultivating gratitude"? Do you picture someone meditating on a beach? Maybe someone taking the time to check out newly blossomed flowers on the way to work? Or perhaps it's someone feeling overwhelmed with anxiety and trying to remind themselves of what's within their control? Cultivating gratitude, like mindfulness, can come in all shapes and sizes.

Cultivating gratitude provides a lens through which you can acknowledge the parts of your life where your needs and desires are being met. It's a way of fully capturing your existence without gaslighting yourself that "nothing is wrong." Gratitude makes space for the good, the bad, and the in between.

One of the benefits of a gratitude list is that you begin to build a practice of looking for things to be grateful for to add to your list, which in turn makes you more present and engaged. This process also helps work against negativity bias. By encouraging you to hold on to the positives in your life as well as the struggles, you can get an accurate picture of what you're experiencing.

Gratitude also helps you identify and follow your values. You are naturally drawn to appreciate or be grateful for what you value in life. So, if you're having difficulty identifying what you're thankful for, consider your values. What do you do that follows your values? What are you grateful for in these parts of your life?

Gratitude can also help raise awareness of your privileges in life. Often our privileges show up on our gratitude list, which can reassure us and offer perspective on where we are relative to others in and out of our communities. What privileges do you hold for which you're grateful?

CALENDARING GRATITUDE

In order to build a practice of gratitude, you'll need to simply do the practice. By writing down your areas of gratitude consistently, you can create a reflective habit to help improve your mental health.

Over the next week, three times a day, reflect on something you are grateful for.

DAY	MORNING: GRATEFUL FOR . . .	MIDDAY: GRATEFUL FOR . . .	EVENING: GRATEFUL FOR . . .
(E.g., Monday)	(E.g., Roof over my head)	(E.g., Conversation with a friend)	(E.g., Delicious dinner)
Monday			
Tuesday			
Wednesday			
Thursday			
Friday			
Saturday			
Sunday			

Don't stop after the week is up. Now that you've experienced reflecting on gratitude three times a day through this exercise, try to engage in this practice on your own moving forward. Over time, try to recognize the benefits of tracking your gratitude.

SHARING GRATITUDE

When you share it with others, gratitude can have an extra layer of pleasure. Use the prompts below to reflect on what it's like to share your appreciation with others.

Person you shared your gratitude with:

_____

What did it feel like to share? (Try to write more than a few words.)

_____

_____

_____

_____

Person you shared your gratitude with:

_____

What did it feel like to share? (Try to write more than a few words.)

_____

_____

_____

_____

Person you shared your gratitude with:

_____

What did it feel like to share? (Try to write more than a few words.)

_____

_____

_____

_____

MATEO'S ANXIOUS ACCEPTANCE

"I hate that I'm this anxious," Mateo blurted out in therapy. He'd been going to weekly therapy for six months after a brutal breakup with a long-term partner. During this time, he had realized many ways his needs weren't being met, and that he wasn't taking care of himself. He also started to cringe and feel ashamed of some of his past choices.

He shared with his therapist that recognizing all the changes he wanted to make was overwhelming, and he felt he couldn't make them fast enough. "Why am I still so anxious? I can't do anything right! I haven't made any progress."

Mateo's therapist playfully replied, "So, you feel exactly the same as you did one year ago?"

"No, I was a mess back then. I reacted to everything and was so anxious I could barely sleep." In his response, he realized he had been using all-or-nothing language while feeling anxious, which only made his anxiety worse.

"Simply name what's happening. Don't add any judgment or editorializing," the therapist suggested.

"I'm feeling anxious," Mateo replied with a sigh, "because I recognize ways I want to change, and I'm not changing as fast as I'd like. It's hard to admit how I treated myself in the past, but it's the only way I can move forward." Eventually, Mateo worked on accepting who he is and where he is in life. It was constant work, but soon enough, he noticed his anxiety lessened the more he admitted that it was sometimes part of his experience.

Practicing Mindfulness

For something as chill and relaxed as mindfulness, people often feel intimidated by the concept. However, mindfulness, meditation, and living in the present moment can help remove many of the anxieties and stresses that men face daily. When you are constantly living in your head, it takes away from your ability to appreciate the present moment. This can cause a lot of anxiety and stress, especially when you are constantly bombarded with negative thoughts.

Mindfulness and meditation can help you learn to focus on your breath and the present moment. This can let you take a step back from your thoughts and emotions and allow you to understand them better. By taking some distance from your thoughts and feelings, accepting them but not following them, you increase self-compassion and reduce stress.

In addition, mindfulness can help you develop a better sense of self-awareness. When you are more aware of your thoughts and emotions, you can understand why you react to certain things in certain ways. Addictions and compulsive behaviors greatly benefit from mindfulness because mindfulness helps you slow down in the moment and take stock of your actions and reactions.

Remember to avoid falling into the trap of expecting perfection in mindfulness. Mindfulness can come in all forms, look like different activities, and take different lengths of time. There is no one right way to practice mindfulness. Whether you do a one-minute silent sit or a seven-day retreat, the point of mindfulness is not to beat your personal record. Instead, find moments of mindfulness by doing things like focusing on the process of washing dishes, holding your attention on a pen, or concentrating on the sounds of nature while taking a hike. Allowing space for mindfulness gives you room to understand yourself better and raise self-awareness.

Overall, mindfulness and meditation can be valuable tools in helping men improve their mental health. They provide a way to disconnect from your negative thoughts and emotions and help you better understand yourself.

MINDFULNESS COMES IN ALL FORMS

As you've learned, you can engage in mindfulness in all sorts of ways. Many of the guys I've spoken to talk about mindfulness as if they need to prepare for a weeklong backpacking trip. However, you can engage in mindfulness any time, and it doesn't require any gear! The point of mindfulness is to be present in the moment, accept what is in front of you, and not try to control your thoughts or emotions.

You can engage in mindfulness while doing the dishes, participating in healthy movement, immersed in creative activities, or during a work meeting. Today, make it a point to engage in some form of everyday mindfulness. It can be for a few seconds or for as many minutes as you desire or are able. What's important is that you make a point to engage in mindfulness.

Identify three ways you will try to engage in mindfulness today and throughout the week.

1. _____
   _____
   _____
   _____

2. _____
   _____
   _____
   _____

3. _____
   _____
   _____
   _____

THOUGHTS ON BY

Now that you're more practiced in mindfulness, begin to work on imagining your thoughts floating by you and then drifting away. This imagery can be helpful in gaining distance from your thoughts and in grounding yourself.

1. Choose a form or shape for your thoughts: (e.g., clouds, sheep, chocolates on a conveyor belt).

2. Now take a current concern and imagine it has taken the form of your chosen shape.

3. Watch it pass by in front of you.

4. Don't try to control its pacing or try to pick it up or force it away. Just let it pass by.

5. When it has passed by, consider adding another concern to the image list and watching it too pass by.

6. Repeat until you feel complete with your mindfulness exercise. Then, if time permits, consider responding to or reflecting on the questions provided.

What was it like to sit and watch your concerns float by?

_____

_____

What is difficult about not interacting with the concerns?

_____

_____

Making Healthy Choices

Influencing and maintaining your mental health involves many small choices in your day-to-day life. But how do you know you're making the "right" choices? It's easy to be overwhelmed with all the advice thrown at you, but the best way to make choices that are right for you is to find those that appeal to you and meet your needs.

Some things that can help improve and maintain your mental health include:

A rich and varied social life. I could just put "social life," but I want you to push yourself to expand your social network and deepen your current friendships and relationships. Try to get out of your comfort zone and join a men's group or strike up a conversation with a trusted friend. Check in with yourself before, during, and after to see how making some changes in this arena impacts you.

Physical activity. This could be traditional exercise or anything that raises your heart rate. Consistent and regular physical activity significantly improves your mental health. Benefits of regular physical exercise include increased blood circulation to the brain, increased neurochemicals like dopamine, reduced stress, improved connection to your body, increased interest in sex, and reduced tiredness, to name a few.

A balanced diet. Note that I am not naming what weight or diet you should have. That decision is ultimately for you and your trusted health providers. However, it's essential to understand how your diet impacts your mental health. With growing research that our mental health is connected to gut health, you can benefit from diets that reduce inflammation-related issues.

Sleep. Sleep is significantly tied to your psychological and emotional well-being. This is a surprise to no one. If you're sleep deprived, it's tough to think clearly or react calmly. You're just raw. By working on your relationship with sleep by knowing what you need to wind down at night and creating the proper environment for rest, you can improve your sleep routine.

A healthy relationship with drugs and alcohol. There are benefits and disadvantages to drugs and alcohol that vary depending on the person, so this is another category where it's essential to find the best relationship for you. Substance abuse and misuse make it hard to access your emotions or find the stability needed to build self-awareness, hold yourself accountable, or make consistent changes you may need. Examine your relationship with alcohol and other drugs to see how it improves your life and what it takes away from you.

These are just some of the domains to consider when making healthy choices. In the following exercises, you'll learn ways to explore and identify the approaches that work for you and how to have a more accepting relationship with yourself.

WHAT HEALTHY CHOICES DO YOU MAKE?

Everyday life is rife with erratic swings of health advice. One year, eggs are a life-saver; the next year, they are guaranteed to stop your heart. Let's not forget about the endless supplements that are marketed to men day after day. However, you get to decide what is healthy for you.

What are you currently doing to maintain your health and connect to your body?

_____

_____

_____

_____

How do these things connect to your values?

_____

_____

_____

_____

How can you start to maintain your health and promote self-care?

_____

_____

_____

_____

How do these things connect to your values?

_____

_____

_____

_____

SO JUDGY

Self-judgment is a common experience for most people. It can be especially diffi-cult for men, who are often socialized to bottle up their emotions and "suck it up." Unfortunately, this can lead to feelings of inadequacy and a negative self-view. This exercise is designed to help you break apart your judgment to understand it better.

1. Keep note of when you judge yourself and input the thought in the table on page 82.

2. Self-judgments are often connected to insecurities or concerns. Take a moment to identify what insecurities or concerns are connected to the corre-sponding judgment.

3. To give yourself perspective, identify what you are doing to address these insecurities or concerns. This can also include acceptance of what cannot be changed or controlled.

4. Take the statement in the first column and reframe it to merely state the facts instead of including your judgmental interpretation. This will allow you to get a clearer perspective of the situation.

5. Try to use all the information gathered to increase self-compassion and move away from judgment.

CONTINUED

JUDGMENTAL THOUGHT ABOUT YOURSELF	CONCERNS CONNECTED TO THE JUDGMENT (E.G., HEALTH, PUNCTUALITY, PERFORMANCE, ETC.)	WHAT THINGS ARE YOU DOING TO ADDRESS THESE CONCERNS?	JUDGMENT REFRAMED AS A PURELY FACTUAL STATEMENT
(E.g., I'm so stupid, I totally messed up the work presentation.)	*(E.g., Intelligence, work performance, job, and financial security)*	*(E.g., Working on my public speaking skills)*	*(E.g., I blanked out at the beginning but after a few minutes I was okay.)*

After completing this exercise, continue to work on being curious about why these patterns show up, and attempt to counteract them with compassion and kindness.

> *When my harsh inner critic shows up, I will acknowledge him, give him a silly name, and let him be on his way. I take away his power over me by not arguing with him.*

Personal Acceptance

Acceptance is not complacency or "giving up." Not only can it be easy to confuse these approaches, but you have also likely seen people misuse the concept of acceptance to avoid conflict. However, this book refers to acceptance as a form of everyday mindfulness to review your surroundings and circumstance and accept what is there. Acceptance doesn't mean agreeing with an experience, co-signing on it, or endorsing it. You can completely accept something while not liking it at the same time. In *Radical Acceptance*, author Tara Brach says, "Radical Acceptance is the willingness to experience ourselves and our lives as it is."

Acceptance allows you to put your energy into the areas of your life that you control. If it helps, think of it as a matter of efficiency. By reserving your energy to focus on parts of yourself and your life that you have control over, you're saving yourself from burnout and despair caused by trying to alter the unalterable. By accepting where you're at in life and what's within your control, paradoxically, you can then make the necessary changes in life for better mental health.

I often hear men reflect on where they are in life with judgment or even disdain. Whether it's related to financial success, career, social-emotional development, or marriage/family planning, it's incredibly easy for you to feel "not enough." Watch out for saying things like "I should" or "I shouldn't." These sayings can indicate self-judgment. Instead, try reframing them into statements of acceptance, and then, if there is anything to change, commit to yourself and others to work on what's within your control.

By now, you should see how treatments like ACT can work for issues around anxiety, shame, trauma, grief, personal development, and more. Stay mindful of when you "'should" all over yourself. If you find yourself saying something like "I shouldn't have this much issue with calming my anxiety down," you can say instead "I'm having a hard time slowing my anxiety down" or "I'm judging myself for having a lot of anxiety right now." What matters is that you're honest and direct with yourself while also taking steps to make choices that will help you stay aligned with your values and needs.

DO SOMETHING YOU ARE GOOD AT

No one is perfect, and everyone has their talents and shortcomings. However, giving yourself permission and time to do something you're good at can improve your mental health. Whether it's a hobby or activity that you enjoy or something you're exceptionally skilled at, doing something that makes you happy is crucial to a fulfilling existence.

So, for this exercise, do something you're good at and use the space provided to log your feelings and reflections.

Activity/hobby:

_____

Describe what you did:

_____

_____

_____

_____

_____

What emotions came up for you before, during, and after?

_____

_____

_____

_____

_____

What did it feel like in your body?

_____

_____

_____

_____

_____

_____

What needs were met in this activity?

_____

_____

_____

_____

_____

_____

How can you use these reflections to build up your confidence?

_____

_____

_____

_____

_____

_____

UNGUILTING YOUR HOBBIES

You've likely experienced the dreaded "hobby turned obligation" trap: You develop a hobby out of pure joy and wonder, even begin to get a knack for it and get more passionate, only to later feel like the activity is a chore. Your once-favorite hobby suddenly looms over you like a guilt-ridden reminder. Obviously, that guilt doesn't inspire anyone to dive back into their passion. Instead, this guilt creates a power struggle between parts of yourself.

For this exercise, choose an activity you now or once enjoyed, then work on identifying the judgments associated with it and write them in the table.

HOBBY	NEED IT MEETS	ASSOCIATED GUILT
(E.g., Painting)	*(E.g., Creativity)*	*(E.g., Worried I'm "wasting" my time being unproductive)*

Filling out this table will help you acknowledge the importance of your own needs and let you pick up a hobby knowing exactly why you are spending your time and resources on this pastime.

Chapter Reflection

In this chapter, you learned about the science behind stress, and aspects of mindfulness like gratitude and acceptance. You also identified new coping skills through exercises and reflective prompts. Before you jump to the next section, give yourself a few moments to sit with what you learned. Identify what emotions or memories were stirred up for you in the process of the workbook. Try to include more than thinking about the chapter or considering what was "interesting." Seek out emotions or physical sensations to inform how you reacted to the contents.

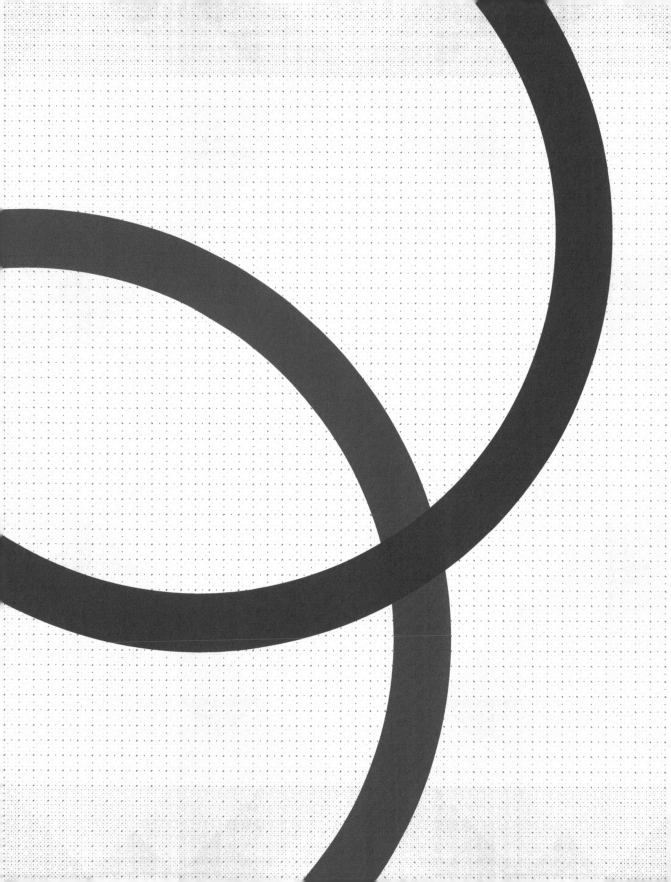

CHAPTER FOUR

SOCIAL WELL-BEING AND MENTAL HEALTH

> *I am allowed to show my true self to others.*
> *Being authentic to who I am is important.*
> *I am enough, and people will see that.*

How You Interact

When considering how you interact with the world, it's easy to go into a categorical "men do this" and "women do that" binary, taking away any nuance or complexity to gender and the gender spectrum. Although there are studies to show that men can often be avoidant with their emotions, a growing number of men are improving their emotional access. The number of men doing so will also increase as more men have healthy expressions of emotions and normalize vulnerable interactions. As you read the descriptors of how men commonly socialize, consider how you do and do not fit into the research and make choices based on your values.

When examining how men interact, some researchers have found that many young men wanted to express themselves emotionally but feared being humiliated or shamed for being vulnerable. Another study found that men often compartmentalize their social groups, aren't sure how to express their feelings, and identify with being independent, which they cited as the reason they didn't socialize. Additional research found that many men in heterosexual relationships relied on their partners for emotional support, which then upheld a public image of emotional independence and stoicism that matches socially prescribed versions of masculinity.

Although these results don't capture all men, they do touch on many reasons why men have difficulty interacting with others. Many men end up lacking practice in expressing themselves due to a fear of vulnerability, yet it wouldn't feel so vulnerable after trying it again and again over time. Meanwhile, there are scores of men who want to be vulnerable but are afraid of humiliation.

In the workplace, research has shown that in general, women interact to establish a social connection, share ideas, and learn from each other, whereas men interact to assert dominance and establish control. In her writing, bell hooks explains how this form of establishing control and dominance also shows up in relationships with friends, family, and significant others. Other examples of goals for interacting can be building community, offering warmth and comfort, or learning. Consider how you approach interactions and relationships and analyze what you want to accomplish in these interactions.

Attachment Styles

Attachment theory is a hot topic in the psychological world, and for good reason. It can explain why some of your relationships are healthy and fulfilling while others are tumultuous and corrosive. Once you understand how you interact with others, you can choose which relationships you'd like to work on adapting.

John Bowlby, a child psychologist, conceptualized attachment as an evolutionary trait to keep infants close to caregivers. In more day-to-day terms, think of attachment as your style of connecting with others. Do you tend to get close to people right away or take a while to warm up? These can indicate your attachment style.

There are three main attachment styles: avoidant, anxious, and secure. Avoidant attachment involves unconscious attempts to create distance from people due to a distrust in others, lack of desire for relationships, or lack of consistent caregivers growing up. Anxious attachment involves a dread or concern that the other person doesn't like or love you, and that relationships won't last. You often need reassurance that things are okay. Lastly, a secure attachment is a style of connection that is calm and certain. You are comfortable being close in relationships and are able to spend time apart without concern. As you read more on attachment styles, consider which styles resonate with you.

KWAME'S ANXIOUS WAITING

After a couple of dates and many text messages, Kwame stopped hearing from Isabella. It felt like it came out of nowhere. "I don't know what to do," he told a friend. "I can't stop thinking about her. I look through our messages to see if I said something wrong or missed something, but nothing comes up." His heart would race, and he would feel a pit in his stomach. Kwame started to beat himself up emotionally. "I came on too strong, I seemed too needy. Did my breath stink?" The more he tried to figure out what was going on, the more his heart raced.

He could feel himself getting worked up from the anxiety, making it almost impossible to stay still. To clear his mind, Kwame went for a run. Running was a hobby he had loved years ago, but he'd left it behind because he started to feel obligated to the routine. The sensation of putting on his old sneakers sparked vivid positive memories of running. He could feel himself begin to breathe a bit easier in relief. As Kwame took off on his run, he worked on watching his thoughts drift by like clouds, so he could visualize letting them go. By the end of his run, he saw on his phone that Isabella had finally responded. Looking at the time stamp, he realized it had only been eight hours since she responded. He decided to use this as a perspective-taking moment rather than beat himself up over "shoulds."

Avoidant Attachment

People with avoidant attachment styles tend to be independent, self-reliant, and uninterested in close relationships. They often avoid intimacy and emotional closeness and may seem distant or aloof. Although more men are known to have an avoidant attachment style, it can affect people of any gender.

Early relationships involving emotionally or physically inconsistent or neglectful caregivers can result in an avoidant attachment style. Furthermore, narcissistic parents can sometimes lead to avoidant attachment. This connection is due to the parent making themselves the center of focus, not only pulling attention and affection from the child but also ensuring that the parent has the upper hand.

People with avoidant attachment style may have difficulty trusting others and feel uncomfortable with intimacy. They might have trouble expressing their emotions and may even suppress their feelings to avoid vulnerability. Although people with avoidant attachment styles can appear to be uninterested in close relationships, they may still crave intimacy and connection.

Underneath their seeming indifference, they may yearn for closeness but feel unable to trust or let down their guard. If you think you might have an avoidant attachment style, it's important to seek out supportive relationships where you feel safe expressing your emotions. By having the experience of expressing your feelings and having them be received with warmth and compassion, you can restructure your attachment style.

Another way to build more secure attachment styles is to identify the reasons behind your distance from others. Then investigate what evidence is and isn't there to back up this concern, or identify what you can accept as a known risk. Some examples can be avoiding a relationship because you don't want to risk getting hurt in a breakup, or stating that dating is "too much drama" because of conflict. Again, self-reflection through therapy or journaling can help you address these concerns.

VALUABLE RELATIONSHIPS

Shared values are often a big reason why people choose their partner. At the same time, you don't need to share every value with your partner. Some differences can be beneficial to each of you and the relationship.

Referring to earlier exercises in the book, what values do you prioritize in relationships?

_____

_____

_____

_____

_____

Why do you prioritize them? What meaning do they have for you?

_____

_____

_____

_____

_____

How do you enact those values?

_____

_____

_____

_____

_____

Anxious Attachment

Anxious attachment style is a term used to describe a condition where a person has difficulty maintaining secure and trusting relationships. People with anxious attachment styles may be preoccupied with the possibility of abandonment or betrayal by their partners and often feel insecure and inadequate in their relationships.

Anxious attachment is characterized by feelings of insecurity, anxiety, and a need for reassurance. Individuals with this type of attachment often have difficulty trusting others, and intimacy can be challenging. Signs that you may have an anxious attachment style include:

- Having difficulty being away from your partner

- Needing constant reassurance

- Being overly sensitive to criticism

- Having a preoccupation with fears of abandonment

Although this type of attachment can be challenging to overcome, some things can be done to build a more secure attachment.

Building more secure attachment involves understanding how you relate to others and shifting patterns that may work against you. Ideally, you would find a secure relationship with someone, which can include a platonic friendship or a working relationship with a therapist. The point is to have an experiential example of someone you feel securely attached to and who you know will be consistent and reliable. This person can model healthy boundaries and communication while you work on your side of the relationship. Try to look at the facts of what's going on in your dynamic, accept what can and can't be changed, and build more coping skills. Track what is currently happening and what you might be reacting to from the past. Your best skill in this process is to slow down in thought, emotion, and action.

As you can see, creating opportunities for intimacy and connection, particularly in relationships with men, can help build trust and slowly reduce fears of abandonment. In addition, seeking professional help to address underlying issues can be beneficial in learning how to develop healthier relationships.

MAPPING OUT RELATIONSHIPS

As you begin to reflect on your relationship styles and habits, take a moment to identify any relationship patterns you have around beginning partnerships.

When starting relationships, do you tend to go slow or dive in fast? Explain what it's like.

_____

_____

_____

_____

_____

What are your expectations within a relationship (e.g., time spent together, support offered each other, etc.)?

_____

_____

_____

_____

_____

What are your core beliefs around building a relationship (e.g., how long until moving in together, monogamous or polyamorous, etc.)?

_____

_____

_____

_____

_____

Secure Attachment

Last, there is secure attachment. Those with secure attachment make up the majority, at 56 percent of the American population. Secure attachment includes:

- Ease of connection with others

- Trusting that the people in your circle are reliable and care for you

- Confidence in your ability to choose trustworthy people

- Comfort being in close relationships or being vulnerable

- Clear and direct communication skills

People with this style tend to come from consistently present and emotionally available families. The experience of this stability offered regular reassurance to their nervous system, helped their view of relationships, and increased their ability to trust others.

Although it may seem like you're absolved of any work in relationships because you're stable and secure, relationships of all kinds need and deserve attention and work. Additionally, suppose you are in a relationship with someone who is anxious or avoidant. In that case, the relationship benefits from you offering more direct communication and checking in with them on how you can support them in the relationship. This does not mean centering the relationship entirely on their needs and wants. However, it does include considering what they are working through and how you can support them without going past your boundaries and values. By offering patience and compassion while recognizing your limits, you can provide a "safe enough" environment for your relationship to flourish and for your partner to feel stable and loved.

WHAT'S YOUR LOVE LANGUAGE?

Dr. Gary Chapman first coined the term "love languages" in his book *The 5 Love Languages: The Secret to Love that Lasts.* In it, he outlines five different ways that people express and receive love: words of affirmation, quality time, receiving gifts, acts of service, and physical touch. The domains he describes can easily be applied to any close relationship between friends, family members, or strangers.

Set aside some time to answer the prompts provided in an effort to learn or better understand your love languages.

When someone buys me a physical gift, I feel:

_____

When someone sets aside time to spend with me, I feel:

_____

When someone compliments me, I feel:

_____

When someone takes care of a chore I've been avoiding, I feel:

_____

When someone hugs or kisses me, I feel:

_____

When I want to show affection, I:

_____

CONTINUED

Are there any differences between how you show love and how you receive love? If so, what do you think they are?

_____

_____

_____

_____

_____

> *I can share space with others without worrying that they will take over or overpower my needs.*

The Effects of Loneliness and Isolation

The feeling of loneliness is something that everyone experiences at different points in their lives. But for some, the sense of isolation and disconnection can be pervasive and all-consuming. When considering loneliness, it's essential to identify that there is social loneliness and emotional loneliness. Social loneliness refers to a lack of a social network, whereas emotional loneliness refers to a lack of an attachment figure. Although everyone has different social needs, a lack of intimacy and connection can profoundly impact one's mental and physical health—especially for men. Studies have shown that feelings of loneliness can lead to an increased risk of depression, anxiety, heart disease, stroke, and sleep disorders. In extreme cases, it can even lead to thoughts of suicide.

Fortunately, there are ways to combat loneliness. Reaching out to family and friends, joining community groups, or seeking professional help are all great options for those struggling with loneliness. The most important thing is to remember that you are not alone in your fight against isolation.

LONELY JIN

Jin is a first-generation American-born man in a big city. He graduated from a good college, has a steady career and a lovely apartment, but feels emotionally unfulfilled and empty. He starts noticing that he often has low energy, is restless at night, and just feels overall down. When talking to his therapist, he is asked about his self-care and about his feelings. Jin gives a long list of solo activities. However, when the therapist mentions socializing, Jin immediately admits he is lacking in that department.

He expresses how awkward it has felt to try to make new friends or even call up old ones. "I don't really know what to say beyond the small talk." The therapist reflects that it is common for adult men to feel lonely and not know how to resolve it. Jin contemplates the word "lonely." He never considered using that word, and in a way, he hates that the word fits his experience so well. "Ugh, 'lonely,'" he tells the therapist. "That's not a word I'd like to use for myself. It sounds so weak and needy."

"It's okay to need help," says the therapist. "It's okay to have needs."

After some more discussion, Jin decides to join his therapist's men's group to get more comfortable talking with and emotionally relating to other men. Over time, he feels himself open up more and more to others and naturally seek out other social events. He learns to access and name his emotions, which helps him identify the kinds of conversations and friendships he wants to have.

What comes to mind when you read Jin's story? What parts of his experience do you relate to? Jin showed not only signs of loneliness but also avoidance. However, as he became more direct with his feelings, he could navigate social situations more easily.

There's also something powerful about using the word "lonely." Through the directness of claiming the vulnerability of being lonely, you accept that you need support, and with that acceptance, you can take action to have your needs met.

FINDING YOUR COMMUNITY

One of the best ways to find your community is through volunteering. Not only are you actively engaged in a task that can help with social anxiety, but you are also more likely to meet others with similar values at the volunteer site.

Use the table below to brainstorm some choices to help find the right one for you.

VOLUNTEER ORGANIZATION	WHAT I WILL DO	WHAT NEED OR VALUE THIS OPPORTUNITY MEETS	WHAT WILL HELP ME TAKE ACTION ON THIS
(E.g., Food bank)	*(E.g., Box and bag food)*	*(E.g., Community, giving back, socializing)*	*(E.g., Setting a deadline to apply)*

DEALING WITH SOCIAL ANXIETY

You may find yourself feeling anxious at the idea of finding community and interacting with others. Try this exercise prior to your next social event or outing.

While you slow down your breathing and relax your muscles, repeat these phrases:

- I can take my time getting comfortable at the event before talking to people.

- I have good stories and jokes to share.

- People want to hear my thoughts.

- I can ask great questions.

- I can leave when I need to do so.

How You Relate to Others

When considering how you relate to others, think about your expectations, hopes, and needs for these connections. What are you trying to achieve or accomplish? Is it warmth and support? Excitement and adrenaline? Maybe it's competition and power? Whatever it might be, it's important to identify the desire and values behind the relationship.

Based on your understanding of relationships through attachment theory, you can see that the attachment framework can be eye-opening to the patterns and dynamics you may find yourself in when relating to others. Your attachment style is one of the most important factors influencing how you relate to others. It affects everything from how you seek intimacy and connection to how you handle conflict and build trust. Generally speaking, people with a more secure attachment style are more able to develop intimacy, connection, and trust with others. They're also more likely to resolve conflict healthily.

On the other hand, people with an anxious or avoidant attachment style may have trouble developing intimacy and connection. They may also tend to avoid conflict or intimacy altogether. Ultimately, your attachment style significantly determines how you interact with the world around you.

Through finding ways to increase healthy connections and relationships, you can fortify your mental health and give yourself the emotional nutrition you deserve. Although you may vary from others in terms of the amount of socializing needed, you are a social animal that needs and deserves some healthy social contact.

One way to identify healthy relationships is to consider how you feel in relation to the other person, and how you feel after your hang out. If you notice that you are feeling aligned and equal with your friend and you leave feeling energized, then this could be considered a positive relationship. However, if you're feeling less than or not enough for the other person based on how they talk to you or how you see yourself compared to them, and if you leave feeling drained, these are signs that you'll benefit from examining what you are getting from this relationship. Although some problematic feelings related to your relationships can be a result of your own anxiety and insecurities, it's great to get some perspective on how the other person engages with your connection as well.

DATING YOURSELF

Although there are plenty of resources for dating ideas when it comes to dating others, there is a need to validate and encourage time with yourself. One of the main principles of self-care is to treat yourself with compassion, comfort, and love; however, there is little guidance on what that would look like. Use the space below to describe your perfect day.

A perfect day to myself would include the following types of activities:

_____

_____

_____

_____

_____

I would eat the following foods:

_____

_____

_____

_____

_____

Some good opportunities to try this in the near future would be (include dates to commit to this action):

_____

_____

_____

_____

_____

THE GOOD FRIENDS

Negativity bias can greatly impact your outlook on life and motivation for change. As a reminder of positive experiences and to highlight what you look for in platonic relationships, take some time to reflect on your positive friendships.

Identify a friendship that has had a positive impact on your life.

_____

How did the friendship begin?

_____

_____

_____

_____

_____

_____

What needs does/did the friendship meet?

_____

_____

_____

_____

_____

_____

_____

What do/did you value in the friendship?

_____

_____

_____

_____

_____

_____

What can you take from your thoughts and observations of the past to implement helpful actions to be used currently?

_____

_____

_____

_____

_____

_____

Developing Strong Friendships

Creating and sustaining genuine friendships is paramount to your mental health. Your friendships with others add spice and comfort to your life through experiences like social interactions, emotional support, playfulness, and validation. You will have many opportunities and situations to create new positive connections throughout your life. Yet, for many, cultivating and maintaining meaningful relationships can feel like a daunting task.

Why do so many men find it challenging to make friends? This is especially true later in life. For some, it is because men are conditioned to believe that they must suffer in silence and cannot admit to any weakness or vulnerability. For others, it is primarily related to not knowing how to deepen a friendship or connection.

Building genuine connections with other men in today's world can be challenging. We are often so busy with work and other obligations that we don't have time to get to know each other. This is a shame because intimacy and connection are important parts of life. We can learn so much about ourselves when we open up to another man and let him into our lives. We can also provide support and understanding that may be difficult to find elsewhere. There are many ways to build genuine connections with other men. One is to make time for each other. Put away your phone, turn off the television, and just talk. Get to know each other's stories, hopes, and dreams.

Another way is to do something together that you both enjoy. This could be working out at the gym, playing a sport, or going for a hike. Doing something together will help you bond and create lasting memories. Let each other know you're excited to hang out together and take turns setting up hangouts. Everyone knows it doesn't feel good to always be the one reaching out. Finally, be supportive of each other. If a friend is struggling, be there for them. Listen without judgment and offer advice if asked. Throughout this chapter, you will have opportunities to reflect on your style of connecting and identify what changes you'd like to make.

FRIEND DATE

There's a lot of modeling for romantic dates but very little representation of going out with a friend to spend time with them and get to know them better. Let's change that!

Choose a friend or family member whom you want to ask out on a friend date:

_____

What do they like to do?

_____

_____

_____

_____

_____

_____

Is there anything that you want to introduce to them (e.g., basketball, virtual reality gaming, cooking)?

_____

_____

_____

_____

_____

_____

CONTINUED

FRIEND DATE CONTINUED

What could be a good specific activity for you to do together?

_____

_____

_____

_____

_____

How will you set it up?

_____

_____

_____

Come back after you've completed the exercise to reflect on your experience here:

_____

_____

_____

_____

_____

_____

FRIENDLY EXPECTATIONS

Everyone holds expectations of friends and relationships based on factors like culture, childhood experiences, social pressures, and explicit agreements. By identifying your expectations, you can get a sense of whether you can get those needs met in a friendship and how to express them. So, what are your expectations in friendships?

_____

_____

_____

_____

_____

_____

_____

_____

_____

_____

_____

_____

Asking for Help

There is a common misconception that asking for help is a sign of weakness for men. This could not be further from the truth. On the contrary, seeking assistance when needed can be a sign of strength and resilience. Asking for help shows that you are willing to take action and find solutions to whatever challenges you may face. It can also build better relationships with the people around you and improve your overall well-being.

As independent and self-reliant as you may feel, there comes a time when you will need to ask for help. You may ask for small favors or continual support. Whatever it may be, asking for help can be challenging for some men. If you fall into this category, you benefit from challenging the stereotype that weak men ask for help. This is likely a profoundly ingrained rule you have for yourself.

If you notice yourself having reactions to being given or needing help, take note of what is happening in the situation and be curious about what is behind the reaction. For example, for some, receiving help feels like they are indebted to the person. This may be related to previous trauma. For others, receiving help makes them feel "not enough" because they can't do it independently.

Do your best to challenge these self-defeating narratives. Not only is it a strength to ask for help, but it is also one to know and accept that you need help. Consider that knowing where your growing edges are and receiving help from others only gives you more time to focus on the areas of your strengths. As an example, by hiring a bookkeeper and payroll specialist, I accept that accounting is not my strength, and I leave myself more time to focus on other parts of my life. The following few exercises will help you understand your relationship to asking for help and give you opportunities to improve these skills.

HOW CAN I BE HELPED?

It can sometimes be challenging to know what type of help to ask for, especially if you're the type to take care of others.

Use the table below to determine what you need support for and how and where you can find it.

WHAT FEELS OVERWHELMING RIGHT NOW?	WHAT NEED OR VALUE IS THIS RELATED TO?	WHAT WOULD BE HELPFUL TO ME RIGHT NOW?	WHO CAN I ASK FOR HELP?
(E.g., Looking for a new job)	*(E.g., Financial stability, sense of pride, reduced stress)*	*(E.g., Connecting with people in my network to find job openings)*	*(E.g., Tim, Xiomara, and Patrice)*

YOUR BIG ASK

Use the information in the previous exercise to decide the who and the what around asking for help. Remember, this doesn't have to be perfect. The goal is to do it regularly, so you'll have many chances to try this approach. The point is to ask for help and see how you feel about the experience.

If you feel like you have no problem asking for help, dig a little deeper. What parts of your life do you feel insecure admitting you need help with? Is it related to finances? Your form at the gym? Sexual advice? Accessing emotions? Flesh out what type of support you could use.

Use the space below to reflect on the experience.

_____

_____

_____

_____

_____

_____

_____

_____

_____

_____

_____

_____

_____

_____

_____

DARRYL'S DILEMMA

Darryl had pride in his connection to his community. He had made a reputation for himself as someone who was "selfless" and "always offered help to others." He brought food to sick friends, gave rides to others, and even volunteered at the local food bank. However, behind this strong sense of community toward others, Darryl also held himself to a rigid expectation of self-reliance and independence.

Darryl was mainly unaware of this paradox. If you brought it up to him, he would give a nervous laugh and change the subject. But this was obvious to his friend Misha. "You almost get mad at people for not asking for help, yet here you are following this gender norm of the strong independent man. You're not practicing what you preach, Darryl. You've got to model the act for others." This wasn't the first time he had received this feedback. Sheepishly, he would say to himself, "They're not wrong," instead of admitting, "They're right."

Darryl agreed to ask for help, and his first attempt was to ask Misha, "What do I even ask for help with?"

She laughed and said, "You've got all these examples of how to ask for help right in front of you. It's not that you don't know. You're out of practice. Create a list of things you've helped others with and see what stands out to you. Then decide who is a good person to ask." Over time, Darryl started to follow this advice, including being gentle with himself for needing help and support from others.

Toxic Behaviors in Relationships

You've likely heard the term "toxic" thrown around, but what does it mean? Can something be okay in one relationship but toxic in another? Understanding the different forms of toxic behavior and what makes them so corrosive to relationships can be incredibly useful.

Toxic behaviors generally revolve around power. These behaviors are conscious or unconscious attempts to control your partner or your relationship, whether you're trying to take power or give all the power over to your partner. This can show up in finances, childcare, decision-making, etc. Such toxic behaviors can corrode your self-esteem and relationship, so much so that a core group of these behaviors have been deemed "The Four Horsemen" by John Gottman. Gottman headed the Gottman Institute, a couples therapy research center that examined couples for over forty years. In his studies, he found that most couples who divorce had displayed one or more of the following behaviors:

Criticism: Frequently putting down your partner's intelligence or character, harming their self-esteem and the relationship

Contempt: Looking down on your partner as if they are beneath you

Defensiveness: An inability to receive feedback without making excuses or lashing out at your partner

Stonewalling: Shutting down communication to avoid conflict out of shame or to punish your partner

It should be no surprise that any of these behaviors will drastically impact a relationship. So, what should you do if they show up? Gottman recommends working on a gentle start-up, wherein you slowly introduce an emotionally difficult topic and use a lot of "I" statements. An example would be "I am feeling a lot of distance between us. Can we take some time to talk about what is going on?" You can also combat toxic behaviors by trying to introduce more gratitude in your relationship. Sharing more gratitude with your partner can encourage you to note the positives more than the negatives in your relationship.

HOLDING YOURSELF ACCOUNTABLE

Change cannot start until you admit your role in the relationship.

    Answer the prompts in this exercise based on the work you've done so far, the feedback you've received from others, and what you know about yourself. The more honest you can be, the closer you will get to truly understanding yourself.

What is a toxic behavior that you know or believe you hold?

_____

_____

_____

_____

_____

_____

_____

What is problematic about this behavior?

_____

_____

_____

_____

_____

_____

_____

CONTINUED

HOLDING YOURSELF ACCOUNTABLE CONTINUED

What can you do to change it?

_____

_____

_____

_____

_____

_____

What can you replace that behavior with?

_____

_____

_____

_____

_____

_____

_____

_____

116   MENTAL HEALTH WORKBOOK FOR MEN

GREEN FLAGS

Although it's incredibly important to identify red flags and other issues to steer clear of in your relationships, it's also useful to name positive aspects to look for and cultivate in relationships. These are values or behaviors that nourish you and make you feel good about your connection to a person.

Take a moment to identify the positive aspects of relationships you prioritize. Feel free to add a few of your own that are not included in the list:

☐ Open communication   ☐ Respect boundaries

☐ Quality time   ☐ Express feelings

☐ Sense of humor   ☐ Listen well

☐ Active sex life   ☐ _____

☐ Playful physical contact   ☐ _____

☐ Actively work on themselves ☐ _____

☐ Stable   ☐ _____

These factors can be used to find friends, teammates, accountability buddies, and romantic partners. Keep these green flags in mind as you consider the types of relationships that nourish your well-being.

Independence and Boundaries

Establishing and holding up boundaries is a life skill that many find challenging. You are not alone if you find yourself struggling to establish your boundaries. Setting these limits can be especially difficult in some kinds of relationships. For example, a part of codependency is difficulty in maintaining boundaries.

Now, "codependency" is a term that holds many meanings for different people. For some, it merely describes a couple spending a lot of time together. Although such behavior might be indicative of codependency, there's much more to the concept than that. Codependency entails a lack of boundaries to the point where feeling different emotions, having different reactions, and even liking different activities can feel like a threat to the security of the relationship. Therefore one, both, or all partners will seek sameness as a form of reassurance or security.

Although sharing many similarities can feel lovely, it is not entirely healthy to consciously or unconsciously disallow differences. Keep in mind that there is a spectrum present. Some sameness and similarities are ideal in a relationship. However, you also want to work toward differentiation where you can be "together but different." Your differences can complement and fortify the relationship instead of being seen as corroding your connection.

Differentiation is an ongoing process of defining yourself, articulating boundaries, and coping with the ambiguous anxiety of potentially getting closer to a partner or separating. By working on your own differentiation, you can identify your own feelings, understand what you need, handle rejection or acceptance, and set needed boundaries.

HEARING "NO"

Sometimes it's hard to handle rejection and hear "no," yet it's a necessary life skill. In this exercise, parse out the types of rejection you fear, what they are related to, and how you can appropriately respond in those scenarios. By identifying these arenas of rejection, you can anticipate potential reactions in order to plan an appropriate response. Consider various scenarios in your life where you may face rejection.

SCENARIO	INSECURITY	SELF-SOOTHING SKILL	RESPONSE
(E.g., Turned down for a date)	*(E.g., Loneliness, unattractiveness)*	*(E.g., Reminder of past positive relationships, self-acceptance affirmations)*	*(E.g., "That's too bad, but thank you for letting me know.")*

Consider different scenarios where this can be applied. It may benefit you to think about low-risk circumstances to try this out with a long-term friend, partner, or family member. Respecting people's boundaries helps everyone in the relationship. Furthermore, by having a plan for hearing no, you may feel more confident working through social anxiety.

BASKING IN BOUNDARIES

Boundaries are integral to establishing mental health. It is important to feel comfortable making boundaries and having them honored. Based on your reading of toxic behaviors, boundaries, and independence, what are some boundaries that you benefit from making in your relationships?

In the table provided, describe what the boundary is, why it's important, and how you can start setting and maintaining the boundary. Remember that setting and maintaining boundaries is a process that can take time, patience, and plenty of reminders. Over time, you will develop more ease and confidence in this approach as you practice.

BOUNDARY	IMPORTANCE	RELATIONSHIP THIS APPLIES TO	HOW YOU CAN START SETTING THE BOUNDARY
(E.g., Not working past 7 p.m.)	(E.g., Preventing burnout, increasing quality time with family)	(E.g., Work, romantic, and family)	(E.g., Scheduling my phone to turn off notifications at 7 p.m.)

> *I can slow down and work on choosing my reactions.*
> *Within that choice is a powerful understanding of myself.*

Chapter Reflection

Throughout this chapter, you learned about and examined your attachment styles, reflected on loneliness and deepening your friendships, and ended by looking at how to set and maintain healthy boundaries within your relationships. You also learned how men are positioned to use relationships to seek and establish power. I encourage you to consider trying to build relationships around sharing resources and building connections.

Furthermore, even though independence and self-sufficiency are excellent qualities, masculinity can encourage us to go too far and lead some men toward isolation and health issues. You can make mindful choices to work toward mental health and wellness through your deeper understanding of yourself and your relationship patterns.

Closing

As you wrap up your time with this book, consider what you've learned about yourself. What aspects of yourself did you develop a deeper understanding about? What will you take away from your time with this book?

I hope that you find yourself with a more refined self-awareness that can help you maintain focus, self-assuredness, and emotional regulation.

Throughout this process, you've explored different ways your mental health can be improved as well as compromised. I encourage you to continue reading and practicing the ideas in this book, including being proactive about your self-care, reaching out for help when needed, and creating a supportive community for yourself. Don't wait! What will you do today to boost your emotional well-being?

It's also important to remember to give yourself permission to slow down, to work on your "second reaction," cherish your boundaries, and operate from your values.

If you want to commit and need the support, email me at contact@davidfkhalili.com with the subject line "Workbook commitment" and tell me what you're committed to doing. I will read and reply to every email.

Be well,
David Khalili

Resources

Books

Acceptance and Commitment Therapy Journal: Prompts and Techniques to Practice Acceptance While Building the Life You Want by Josie Valderrama, a clinical psychologist. This journal offers a fantastic, guided approach to implementing ACT into your reflective practice.

The Jealousy Workbook: Exercises and Insights for Managing Open Relationships by Kathy Labriola, therapist and RN. This workbook was created to help the reader understand and work through their own jealousy.

Polysecure: Attachment, Trauma and Consensual Nonmonogamy by Jessica Fern. Whether you're polyamorous or not, this book offers a refreshing lens into attachment theory and relationships. Take an in-depth look at your attachment and learn new ways to approach your relationship.

The Power of Attachment: How to Create Deep and Lasting Intimate Relationships by Diane Poole Heller, PhD. This deep-dive assessment of attachment styles also includes disorganized attachment.

In the Realm of the Hungry Ghosts: Close Encounters with Addiction by Gabor Maté, MD. This book offers a refreshing and compassionate look at addiction, examining the connection between trauma and addiction.

Sex Worriers: A Mindfully Queer Guide to Men's Anxiety around Sex and Dating by David Khalili, LMFT. This workbook focuses on men overwhelmed by anxiety about sex, dating, or relationships. It includes erotic mindfulness exercises to align your nervous system with your sexual response.

The Will to Change: Men, Masculinity, and Love by bell hooks. This book is a powerful examination of masculinity and men's access to love. The text offers a transformational view of masculinity by offering differing perspectives on relationships and love.

Online

Embrace-Autism.com. A resource and assessment website focused on normalizing and supporting those with neurodiversity. Take self-guided assessments designed by autistic researchers and learn how to work with neurodiversity.

GoodMenProject.com. A thorough website including articles, research, resources, and programming for increasing emotional and social support to men.

OpenPathCollective.org. Directory for affordable in-person and online therapists in the United States.

Other

Crisis Text Line. Text "HOME" to 741741. Crisis support via a national text line. The responders will offer a supportive place to text and connect you to the appropriate resources.

Substance Abuse and Mental Health Services Administration Helpline. Call 1-800-662-HELP (4357). National free hotline for individuals and friends or family members of those facing mental health and/or substance use disorders.

References

Agius, M., and C. Goh. "The Stress-Vulnerability Model; How Does Stress Impact on Mental Illness at the Level of the Brain. . . . And What Are the Consequences?" *European Psychiatry* 25, S1 (June 2010): 1591. doi:10.1016/s0924-9338(10)71572-8.

Bader, Ellyn, Peter T. Pearson, and Judith D. Schwartz. *Tell Me No Lies: How to Face the Truth and Build a Loving Marriage*. New York: St. Martin's Press, 2000.

Brach, Tara. *Radical Acceptance: Embracing Your Life with the Heart of a Buddha*. New York: Random House Publishing Group, 2004.

Braund, Taylor A., Donna M. Palmer, Gabriel Tillman, Heidi Hanna, and Evian Gordon. "Increased Chronic Stress Predicts Greater Emotional Negativity Bias and Poorer Social Skills but Not Cognitive Functioning in Healthy Adults." *Anxiety, Stress, & Coping* 32, no. 4 (July 2019): 399–411. doi:10.1080/10615806.2019.1598555.

Bremner, J. Douglas. "Does Stress Damage the Brain?" *Biological Psychiatry* 45, no. 7 (April 1999): 797–805. doi:10.1016/s0006-3223(99)00009-8.

Carhart-Harris, Robin L., and Guy M. Goodwin. "The Therapeutic Potential of Psychedelic Drugs: Past, Present, and Future." *Neuropsychopharmacology* 42, no. 11 (April 2017): 2105–13. doi:10.1038/npp.2017.84.

Chapman, Gary D. *The Five Love Languages: How to Express Heartfelt Commitment to Your Mate*. Chicago: Northfield Publishing, 2004.

Chapman, Gary D. *The 5 Love Languages: The Secret to Love that Lasts*. Chicago: Northfield Publishing, 1992.

Chen, Quanjing, Haichuan Yang, Brian Rooks, Mia Anthony, Zhengwu Zhang, Duje Tadin, Kathi L. Heffner, and Feng V. Lin. "Autonomic Flexibility Reflects Learning and Associated Neuroplasticity in Old Age." *Human Brain Mapping* 41, no. 13 (September 2020):. 3608–19. doi:10.1002/hbm.25034.

Chiesa, Alberto, Raffaella Calati, and Alessandro Serretti. "Does Mindfulness Training Improve Cognitive Abilities? A Systematic Review of Neuropsychological Findings." *Clinical Psychology Review* 31, no. 3 (April 2011): 449–64. doi:10.1016/j.cpr.2010.11.003.

Cleary, Anne. "Death Rather than Disclosure: Struggling to Be a Real Man." *Irish Journal of Sociology* 14, no. 2 (December 2005): 155–76. doi:10.1177/079160350501400209.

Corns, Jennifer. "Rethinking the Negativity Bias." *Review of Philosophy and Psychology* 9, no. 3 (September 2018): 607–25. doi.org/10.1007/s13164-018-0382-7.

Côté, Stéphane. "A Social Interaction Model of the Effects of Emotion Regulation on Work Strain." *Academy of Management Review* 30, no. 3 (July 2005): 509–30. doi:10.5465/amr.2005.17293692.

Cozzarelli, Catherine, Joseph A. Karafa, Nancy L. Collins, and Michael J. Tagler. "Stability and Change in Adult Attachment Styles: Associations with Personal Vulnerabilities, Life Events, and Global Construals of Self and Others." *Journal of Social and Clinical Psychology* 22, no. 3 (June 2005): 315–46. doi:10.1521/jscp.22.3.315.22888.

de Souza-Talarico, Juliana Nery, Marie-France Marin, Shireen Sindi, and Sonia J. Lupien. "Effects of Stress Hormones on the Brain and Cognition: Evidence from Normal to Pathological Aging." *Dementia & Neuropsychologia* 5, no. 1 (January 2011): 8–16. doi:10.1590/S1980-57642011DN05010003.

Firth, Joseph, Nicola Veronese, Jack Cotter, Nitin Shivappa, James R. Hebert, Carolyn Ee, Lee Smith, et al. "What Is the Role of Dietary Inflammation in Severe Mental Illness? A Review of Observational and Experimental Findings." *Frontiers in Psychiatry* 10 (May 2019): 350. doi:10.3389/fpsyt.2019.00350.

Fyfe, Alastair Colin. "Emotional Disclosure: Rethinking the Ways Masculinity Impacts the Willingness to Be Vulnerable." *2021 Psychology: Concentration in Clinical Psychology Masters Theses.* San Francisco State University. May 2021. doi:10.46569/20.500.12680/5t34sr341.

Garlick, Dennis. "Understanding the Nature of the General Factor of Intelligence: The Role of Individual Differences in Neural Plasticity as an Explanatory Mechanism." *Psychological Review* 109, no. 1 (January 2002): 116–36. doi:10.1037/0033-295x.109.1.116.

Gottman, John. *Why Marriages Succeed or Fail: And How You Can Make Your Marriage Last.* New York: Simon & Schuster, 1995.

Graham, Louis F., Robert E. Aronson, Tracy Nichols, Charles F. Stephens, and Scott D. Rhodes. "Factors Influencing Depression and Anxiety among Black Sexual Minority Men." *Depression Research and Treatment* 2011 (September 2011): 1–9. doi:10.1155/2011/587984.

Hanson, Rick, and Forrest Hanson. *Resilient: How to Grow an Unshakable Core of Calm, Strength, and Happiness.* New York: Harmony Books, 2018.

Harris, Dan. *10% Happier: How I Tamed the Voice in My Head, Reduced Stress without Losing My Edge, and Found Self-Help That Actually Works—A True Story.* New York: HarperCollins, 2019.

Hart, Carl. *High Price: A Neuroscientist's Journey of Self-Discovery That Challenges Everything You Know about Drugs and Society.* New York: Harper Perennial, 2014.

Harvard Health Publishing. "Understanding the Stress Response: Chronic Activation of This Survival Mechanism Impairs Health." Harvard Medical School. July 6, 2020. health.harvard.edu/staying-healthy/understanding-the-stress-response.

Helbich, Marco. "Mental Health and Environmental Exposures: An Editorial." *International Journal of Environmental Research and Public Health* 15, no. 10 (October 2018): 2207. doi:10.3390/ijerph15102207.

hooks, bell. *The Will to Change: Men, Masculinity, and Love.* New York: Washington Square Press, 2005.

Hughto, Jaclyn M., Emily K. Quinn, and Michael S. Dunbar. "Prevalence and Co-occurrence of Alcohol, Nicotine, and Other Substance Use Disorder Diagnoses among US Transgender and Cisgender Adults." *JAMA Network Open* 4, no. 2 (February 2021). doi:10.1001/jamanetworkopen.2020.36512.

Khalili, David F. *Sex Worriers: A Mindfully Queer Guide to Men's Anxiety around Sex and Dating.* Self-published, 2021.

Khalsa, Dharma Singh. "Stress, Meditation, and Alzheimer's Disease Prevention: Where the Evidence Stands." *Journal of Alzheimer's Disease* 48, no. 1 (August 2015): 1–12. doi:10.3233/JAD-142766.

Kumpfer, Karol. "Factors and Processes Contributing to Resilience: The Resilience Framework." In *Resilience and Development: Positive Life Adaptations*, ed. Meyer D. Glantz and Jeannette L. Johnson. New York: Kluwer Academic/Pienum Publishers, 1999.

Leaper, Campbell. "Influence and Involvement in Children's Discourse: Age, Gender, and Partner Effects." *Child Development* 62, no. 4 (August 1991): 797–811. doi:10.2307/1131178.

Levine, Amir, and Rachel S. F. Heller. *Attached: The New Science of Adult Attachment and How It Can Help You Find—and Keep—Love.* New York: Penguin Random House, 2011.

Li, Xiaoling, Meicui Chen, Zhicui Yao, Tianfeng Zhang, and Zengning Li. "Dietary Inflammatory Potential and the Incidence of Depression and Anxiety: A Meta-Analysis." *Journal of Health, Population, and Nutrition* 41, no. 1 (May 2022): 24. doi:10.1186/s41043-022-00303-z.

Luders, Eileen. "Exploring Age-Related Brain Degeneration in Meditation Practitioners." *Annals of the New York Academy of Sciences* 1307, no. 1 (January 2014): 82–8. doi:10.1111/nyas.12217.

Martin, Lisa A., Harold W. Neighbors, and Derek M. Griffith. "The Experience of Symptoms of Depression in Men vs Women: Analysis of the National Comorbidity Survey Replication." *JAMA Psychiatry* 70, no. 10 (October 2013): 1100–6. doi:10.1001/jamapsychiatry.2013.1985.

Mason, E. S. "Gender Differences in Job Satisfaction." *The Journal of Social Psychology* 135, no. 2 (April 1995): 143–51. doi:10.1080/00224545.1995.9711417.

McKenzie, Sarah K., Sunny Collings, and Jo River. "Masculinity, Social Connectedness, and Mental Health: Men's Diverse Patterns of Practice." *American Journal of Men's Health* 12, no. 5 (April 2018): 1247–61. doi:10.1177/1557988318772732.

Murphy, Sherry L., Jiaquan Xu, Kenneth D. Kochanek, Sally C. Curtin, and Elizabeth Arias. "Deaths: Final Data for 2015." *National Vital Statistics Reports* 66, no. 6 (November 2017): 1–75. pubmed.ncbi.nlm.nih.gov/29235985.

Newberg, Andrew B., Mijail Surruya, Nancy Wintering, Aleezé Sattar Moss, Diane Reibel, and Daniel A. Monti. "Meditation and Neurodegenerative Diseases." *Annals of the New York Academy of Sciences* 1307, no. 1 (January 2014): 112–23. doi:10.1111/nyas.12187.

Oliffe, John L., Mary T. Kelly, Joan L. Bottorff, Joy L. Johnson, and Sabrina T. Wong. "'He's More Typically Female Because He's Not Afraid to Cry': Connecting Heterosexual Gender Relations and Men's Depression." *Social Science & Medicine* 73, no. 5 (September 2011): 775–82. doi:10.1016/j.socscimed.2011.06.034.

Patel, Jainish, and Prittesh Patel. "Consequences of Repression of Emotion: Physical Health, Mental Health, and General Well Being." *International Journal of Psychotherapy Practice and Research* 1, no. 3 (February 2019): 16–21. doi:10.14302/issn.2574-612x.ijpr-18-2564.

Pyke, Robert E. "Sexual Performance Anxiety." *Sexual Medicine Reviews* 8, no. 2 (April 2020): 183–90. doi:10.1016/j.sxmr.2019.07.001.

Real, Terrence. *Us: Getting Past You & Me to Build a More Loving Relationship.* New York: Rodale Books, 2022.

Reiff, Collin M., Elon E. Richman, Charles B. Nemeroff, Linda L. Carpenter, Alik S. Widge, Carolyn I. Rodriguez, Ned H. Kalin, et al. "Psychedelics and Psychedelic-Assisted Psychotherapy." *American Journal of Psychiatry* 177, no. 5 (February 2020): 391–410. doi:10.1176/appi.ajp.2019.19010035.

Rowe, John W., and Robert L. Kahn. *Successful Aging.* New York: Dell Publishing, 1998.

Rowland, David L., and Jacques J. D. M. van Lankveld. "Anxiety and Performance in Sex, Sport, and Stage: Identifying Common Ground." *Frontiers in Psychology* 10 (July 2019): 1615. doi:10.3389/fpsyg.2019.01615.

Sharma, Ashish, Vishal Madaan, and Federick D. Petty. "Exercise for Mental Health." *Primary Care Companion to the Journal of Clinical Psychiatry* 8, no. 2 (January 2006): 106. doi:10.4088/pcc.v08n0208a.

Substance Abuse and Mental Health Services Administration, Center for Behavioral Health Statistics and Quality. *Treatment Episode Data Set (TEDS): 2004–2014. National Admissions to Substance Abuse Treatment Services.* BHSIS Series S-84, HHS Publication No. (SMA) 16-4986. Rockville, MD: Substance Abuse and Mental Health Services Administration, 2016.

Tangney, June Price, Jeff Stuewig, and Debra J. Mashek. "Moral Emotions and Moral Behavior." *Annual Review of Psychology* 58, no. 1 (February 2007): 345–72. doi:10.1146/annurev.psych.56.091103.070145.

Terry, Natalie, and Kara Gross Margolis. "Serotonergic Mechanisms Regulating the GI Tract: Experimental Evidence and Therapeutic Relevance." *Handbook of Experimental Pharmacology* 239 (December 2016): 319–42. doi:10.1007/164_2016_103.

Torrey, E. Fuller, Beata M. Barci, Maree J. Webster, John J. Bartko, James H. Meador-Woodruff, and Michael B. Knable. "Neurochemical Markers for Schizophrenia, Bipolar Disorder, and Major Depression in Postmortem Brains." *Biological Psychiatry* 57, no. 3 (February 2005): 252–60. doi:10.1016/j.biopsych.2004.10.019.

Valderrama, Josie. *Acceptance and Commitment Therapy Journal: Prompts and Techniques to Practice Acceptance While Building the Life You Want.* Oakland, CA: Rockridge Press, 2022.

Weiss, Robert S. *Loneliness: The Experience of Emotional and Social Isolation.* Cambridge, MA: MIT Press, 1975.

Wichstrøm, Lars., Anna Emilie Borgen, and Silje Steinsbekk. "Parental Personality Disorder Symptoms and Children's Social Skills: A Prospective Community Study." *European Child & Adolescent Psychiatry* (March 2022). doi:10.1007/s00787-022-01965-0.

World Health Organization. "Burn-out an 'Occupational Phenomenon': International Classification of Diseases." May 28, 2019. who.int/news/item/28-05-2019-burn-out-an-occupational-phenomenon-international-classification-of-diseases.

Yanguas, Javier, Sacramento Pinazo-Henandis, and Francisco José Tarazona-Santabalbina. "The Complexity of Loneliness." *Acta Biomedica: Atenei Parmensis* 89, no. 2 (June 2018): 302–14. doi:10.23750/abm.v89i2.7404.

Index

Environmental stressors, 2
Evidence-based practices, 10

F

Feelings. *See* Emotions
Fight, flight, freeze, or fawn
    mode, 33, 65
The 5 Love Languages (Chapman), 97
Friendships, 104–109

G

Goal setting, 14–15
Gottman, John, 114
Gratitude, 72–75
Green flags, 117
Grief, 24
Grit, 46
Guilt, 36, 86

H

Hanson, Rick, 46
Hart, Carl, 62
Healthy choices, 78–80
Help, asking for, 109–113
Hobbies, 84–86
hooks, bell, 2

I

Interactions with others, 89–90
Irritability, 4, 29–32
Isolation, 5, 98–99

J

Joy, finding, 67

K

Kabat-Zinn, Jon, 10

L

Learned helplessness, 11–12
Loneliness, 5, 98–99
Love languages, 97–98

M

Melancholy, 39
Memories, positive, 67
Mental health
  benefits of good, 8
  concerns for men, 4–7
  elements of, 1–2
  environmental factors, 2
  vs. mental illness, 3
  physical health and, 9
  treatment modalities, 10–12
Mental illness, 3
Mindfulness
  about, 10–11
  practicing, 76–78
Mindfulness-based stress reduction, 10
Mood tracking, 7

N

Negativity bias, 53–54, 104
Nervousness, 33. *See also* Anxiety
Neurochemicals, 18, 28–29
Neuroplasticity, 53

P

Performance anxiety, 33, 34
Physical activity, 79
Physical health, 9
Positive psychology, 11–12, 23
Post-traumatic stress disorder
    (PTSD), 56
Pressure to perform, 4

Progress tracking, 13
Psychological mental health
  benefits of good, 8
  elements of, 1
  social conditioning and, 51–52

R

Radical Acceptance (Brach),
    24, 83
Real, Terrence, 36
Rejection, 119
Relationships
  beginning, 95
  green flags, 117
  healthy, 101–102
  toxic behaviors in, 113–116
Resiliency, 45–46

S

Sadness, 39–42
Secure attachment, 90, 96
Self-care, 103
Self-compassion, 38
Self-improvement, as a
    process, 3
Self-judgment, 81–82
Seligman, Martin, 11
Shame, 36–38, 45
"Shoulding," 24, 83, 91
Sleep routines, 79
"Soaking," 23
Social anxiety, 101
Social conditioning, 51–52
Social loneliness, 98
Social networks, 79

Social well-being
  benefits of good, 8
  community-building, 100
  elements of, 1
  friendships, 104–109
  interactions with others, 89–90
  relating to others, 101–102
Stereotypes, effects of harmful, 9, 43
Stonewalling, 114
Stress, 65–70
Substance abuse, 5, 17–18, 79. *See also*
    Addiction

T

Thoughts and thinking
  distancing from distracting, 63
  labeling, 71
  mindfulness for, 78
  social conditioning and, 51–52
Toxic behaviors, 113–116
Trauma
  and mental illness, 3
  responses, 55–56
  unresolved, 5
Treatment modalities, 10–12

V

Valderrama, Josie, 11
Values, 61–62, 93
Volunteering, 100

W

The Will to Change (hooks), 2
Window of tolerance, 56
World Health Organization, 5

Acknowledgments

Thank you to those in my life who cheered me on and shared their encouragement for my thoughts and purpose. To those who helped me create the book, including editors and those close to me, I can't thank you enough. Much gratitude to Mo Mozuch and Charlie Duerr for their support and guidance while creating this book.

About the Author

 David Khalili is a licensed marriage and family therapist and board-certified sexologist. He founded and operates Rouse Relational Wellness, a boutique mental health wellness center in San Francisco focused on sex and relationship therapy emphasizing anxiety, polyamory, multicultural relationships, and trauma survivors. You can learn more about David and his work at DavidFKhalili.com.